Eat More Raw

A Guide to Health and Sustainability

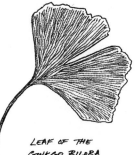

LEAF OF THE
GINKGO BILOBA
TREE — WONDERFUL
PROPERTIES & CAN
OFTEN BE HARVESTED
FROM PUBLIC PARKS!

by Steve Charter

A Simple Living Series Book

Published in the UK by:

Permanent Publications

Hyden House Limited, The Sustainability Centre, East Meon, Hampshire GU32 1HR

Tel: 01730 823 311

Fax: 01730 823 322

Overseas: (international code +44 - 1730)

Email: enquiries@permaculture.co.uk

Web: www.permaculture.co.uk

Text copyright © 2003 Steve Charter.

First published 2004

Reprinted 2006

Designed and typeset by John Adams

Printed by Antony Rowe Ltd., Eastbourne, East Sussex.

Printed on paper from a 100% sutainable source.

British Library Cataloguing - in - Publication Data.
A catalogue record for this book is available from the British Library.

ISBN 1 85623 024 4

Front cover photograph: John Adams
Back cover photograph: Aranya

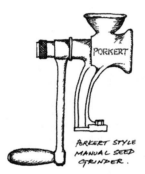

PORKERT STYLE
MANUAL SEED
GRINDER.

The Author

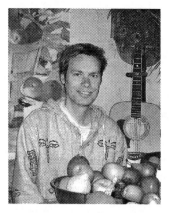

My home now is an ecological vegan raw food forest garden community called Ecoforest in southern Spain, but it hasn't always been like this... as my background and life (so far) are a bit of a mix.

I grew up in deeply middle class west Surrey (England), close to the Hampshire border, with the good fortune of having parents who created a large and beautiful garden to play in. I went to comprehensive school, college and then on to university with no idea whatsoever of what I was doing with my life. Seven average O levels, three average A levels, one very average degree and a whole lot of cricket in between! At 22 I found myself working, of all things, for a small steel trading company, which lasted for six years. This was actually a really good education, and confidence building experience – I learnt a lot from the people I worked with, in England and in the 3 months I worked in the USA.

During that time I started waking up. This accelerated rapidly at 25 when I started to meditate and explore Buddhist thinking, as a practical and compassionate philosophy in life. So, after six years at 28, I quit my 'good job', with company car and a 'good mortgage', packed up my southern lifestyle (which did include going to CND demos, and being a Green Party member by the way) and went off to do an MA in Environmental Planning in Nottingham, ten years to the day after starting my first degree. The difference was that this time I knew what I was doing and why I was doing it!

After 2 years I found I'd won the course prize with my dissertation on 'Planning for Sustainability?', with part time lecturing following over the next three years. I also set up a University Green Society and was one of two student reps on the University Environment Committee, whilst also attending Greenpeace and Green Party meetings in the city. Life had become busy, but far more fun and much more purposeful. With my MA complete I went to work on the Local Agenda 21 (sustainable development) strategy within Leicester Environment City – a European Union funded post to develop a model approach to Agenda 21 for cities. I did that from 1993 to late 1995, which means that I turned out to be one of the first people in Britain (and therefore the world!) to work on Agenda 21 as a job. Despite working with a good team, I left Leicester disillusioned with the LA21 process and the political realities of greenwash. The best project I was involved in there was outside of my work trying to set up a community garden in an area that really needed and deserved it. But the politicians and council officers had other priorities, so they did nothing to make that particularly inspiring green community project happen in so called Leicester Environment City!

During my time in Leicester I grew to see that the grass-roots was where the moves towards real sustainability were coming from. So I then got more into permaculture by doing an amazing, life-changing 2 week permaculture design course in September '94 at Turner's Field near Glastonbury in Somerset. I also discovered about raw food nutrition on that course.

A year later I left Leicester and moved down to Devon to establish a shared raw food house with five others that became the centre for the FRESH Network and the information and event centre for the raw food community of the UK for 18 months. This was a fascinating, challenging and extraordinary time, that deserves a book in itself – there was far more to it than just the raw food!

As an example, the kinds of explorations that went on at this time later led to a fully monitored and utterly unique five day sleep deprivation experiment with Manchester Metropolitan University! This experiment was organised and overseen by the respected and fairly well known sports psychologist, Professor Dave Collins. Well, yes, it was indeed quite an adventure. And the results over the five days are still unique for any sleep deprivation experiment any where in the world (i.e. on average we experienced *improved* dexterity, physical agility, mental acuity, and a generally cheery state of affairs). These results were much more of a surprise for Professor Collins and his research colleagues than for Tony and myself, who did the staying awake! The secret? Well, it's the only such experiment to have ever involved long term raw fooders... so possibly that may have a little something to do with the unique results.

Around the time of the shared raw house in Devon I connected up with the Plants for a Future project, which was very positive, and I met Robert Hart for the first time. I also did lots of writing and personal research on a whole range of issues (particularly sustainability/unsustainability and their relationship to human patterns – social patterns, economic patterns, patterns of civilisation and consciousness, etc.), as well as running a series of local permaculture courses with my good friend Simon Shakespeare, and setting up a local permaculture network – The Exe Valley Permaculture Network.

I then had some interesting times, living in various places in Somerset, including a wonderful six months at Turner's Field, living there with my good friend Ann Morgan and an enigmatic northern Irish chap called Louis. I moved from Turner's Field after two months of connection with possibly the most extraordinary place and people I have ever visited – Tiaia in western Eire. This threw me into a state of creative yet somewhat disconcerting chaos. And after connecting with this awesomely beautiful, barefoot, place of 'ecotarian' paradise gardening, nine months of being barefoot followed... which despite what you may think was fantastically enlivening, and not difficult most of the time (I admit I wasn't doing any conventional work at that time!). I eventually brought the 100% barefoot phase to a close for a variety of reasons; primarily because in this culture I found that living outside of community situations it just gets too tiring trying to live in ways that don't fit the norm. It was also heading for winter!

Another reason for me putting my boots back on was that at that time I started regularly visiting Robert Hart travelling by motorbike... which doesn't really suit bare feet! It was the winter about a year before Robert died, and I was working with him trying to produce the book he so desperately wanted to write. That got very difficult because of my own penniless circumstances at the time, my over-stretched commitments elsewhere, and because of Robert's variable health. Over time though I have persisted with that work because it has felt so important. It is about the peaceful and positive ecological revolution, and the practical tools, ideas and philosophies which we all need to implement and accelerate now! So that's one for you to look forward to I hope.

In the last few years I've been focusing on keeping my sometimes bare sometimes very much shoed feet in the grass roots stuff whilst also re-connecting with the more establishment world of sustainability and Agenda 21. On the grass roots side, with a wide group of others, and two other trustees in particular, I have been setting up Ecoforest. This is an ecological vegan raw food forest garden community and eco-education project in Spain, with an associated UK based Trust – see Appendix 3. This is going really well, getting fantastically positive feedback from our visitors, and growing all the time. So I now find that I am a Trustee and Secretary of The Eco Forest Garden Trust, and most of the time live in a wonderful place with some fantastic and beautiful people. I am also a Trustee of Forest Inspirations.

During exactly the same period of time I have also been re-entering the weird world of local government sustainability work. In 1999 I set up a community enterprise called Somerset Sustainable Housing with a highly skilled and motivated timber framer friend, and completed The Somerset Sustainable Housing Study. As a result of this work, which received a good amount of very positive feedback, in 2000 I was employed for six months as consultant by South Somerset District Council to initiate and implement the pioneering South Somerset Sustainable Construction Strategy. As well as having a significant influence on planning work, social housing, community buildings and the council's own buildings, this lead to the establishment of the unique Somerset Trust for Sustainable Development – see Appendix 3. The Trust works as a training and educational organisation, a consultancy, and an ethical community based developer that only undertakes sustainable construction projects. The Trust's mission is 'to make sustainable const-ruction the norm, rather than the exception by 2010'. I have now relinquished my role as Research Director of the Trust. For those that are quite rightly concerned about the ecological and atmospheric effects of air travel, whilst my life is currently split between Spain and England, I definitely avoid flying, and travel mostly by ferry in a shared vehicle. Most of my work for the Trust is now writing guides to sustainable construction (e.g. for school buildings), which I can do on a remote basis.

I have experienced and enjoyed both great change and great diversity in my life so far. Going from being barefoot to wearing a suit 'n' tie again and working with Councils as a consultant within one year (1999 - 2000) was interesting and involved a bit of a weird reality shift. Both have been very positive experiences, although the latter has probably been a little harder and not quite as much fun as the former! But it does show that such things are possible.

My major writing project of the last few years has been *The Earth Dwellers' Guide to Sustainability*, and following a period where it has been sitting in a lay-by waiting for the right bus to come along I now know it's time to get The Guide moving again. With the confusion of 'Millennium Fever' out of the way, and the ripple effects of Earth Summit III in 2002 I feel there is a good chance that more people will start waking up to what sustainability issues really imply for our lives... and they may even start to realise that sustainable development and sustainability are not the same thing, and that the former may not in fact be the best means to achieve the latter. Get the book if you want to know more!

In the Guide I present the issues in an open way, looking at the issues from a variety of perspectives. There's the main book, *The Earth Dwellers' Guide to Sustainability* which includes an introduction and a major section on the background detail of sustainability and sustainable development. Then there are six inter-related chapters on key topics – the conventional 'big three' of Economics, Society and Environment, and an alternative yet equally relevant 'big three' of Civilisation, Consciousness and the Individual. To conclude the book, and to start change in the reader's life, there is then a section on 'Solutions and Conscious Responses'. I have self-published these separately in various forms over the last few years, and have got only positive feedback from my readers. But the Guide doesn't quite fit the normal publishing pigeon holes, so it has taken a while for it to spread its wings and fly.

The intention is that a) people can see the inter-connectedness of the issues, and b) they can judge for themselves and draw their own conclusions. I had a lot of encouragement in the early days of writing from The Oakwood Trust; the UK 'branch' of Fritjof Capra's Elmwood Trust in the USA, which promotes ecoliteracy and an understanding of interconnectedness. *The Earth Dwellers' Guide* is finally maturing and it should be ready to make its own way in the big wide world soon.

So since September 1994 I have maintained a 90-100% raw diet (mainly 95%+), with many periods of being 100% raw within that time. I have been vegan since 1991, and vegetarian since 1988. I have not had any ongoing problems of slipping back into the numerous plates and pans of 'normal' cooked food that surround me in life, and have enjoyed excellent health and plenty of mental and physical energy throughout.

However, at times in my raw journey I have had a patchy and difficult relationship with what is undoubtedly a hard drug – namely coffee! (Yes, ok, the drug is caffeine, I know.) Man! It's only when you come off such things that you realise how powerful an effect these highly profitable, legal drugs have (alcohol and nicotine being the two other obvious ones). This kind of realisation often happens when you first go raw – your eyes are opened! For me, coffee has been very strongly associated with work, and sitting at a PC doing work that I felt was important but which I did not really want to be doing. Coffee has been very effective in shutting down my sensitivities when doing this work, whilst also living in a world that often feels harsh, destructive and uncaring. This has perhaps been useful at times as a survival strategy, but coffee definitely has a harsh effect on one's emotions and nervous system, and its addictive quality has helped me maintain my inner conflict about using it. When I'm drinking coffee I am a different person – more intense and mentally energised, but I am not at all my true, natural self. So whilst I did not slip back into plates and pans of cooked food and have had no desire to do so, on and off and for varying lengths of time I was swimming around in mugs and jugs of coffee for far too long! And that has kept me working in areas that are basically positive, but which I have felt for years are only dealing with the symptoms and not the underlying causes of ill-health, unsustainable lifestyles and the unfulfilled lives that so many people lead.

Most of these years, having discovered raw food and the power and beauty of permaculture at the same time on my 2 week Permaculture Design course back in '94, I have been fortunate generally to live in places where either I could quickly create a pretty good salad garden, or where one already existed – this has been really important. Throwing in a few seeds and a special selection of perennials has a wonderful effect – it creates food! So I've enjoyed the delights of a vibrant and varied green salad most evenings since late '94, with the joys of Turner's Field and Tiaia salads being the peaks of that particular experience! Getting those really vibrant greens in almost every day has been 'vital'.

And as for this book, well it's an outcome of all those experiences, and it results as much from the people I've met along the way, their work and the inspiration they have provided, as it does from my own efforts. So I thank you all, my friends, and I hope that this book does as much good for the reader as the experiences I've described above have done for the writer!

Have fun and don't be afraid to adventure with your life folks – I can tell you from experience that living a healthier and much more sustainable life can be a whole lot of fun!

Steve Charter

Acknowledgements

I express great thanks to... Robert Hart (1913-2000) for his vision, wisdom and humility, for encouraging me so much to write this book, for his contribution to it and for being such an inspiration to so many; Tony Wright for his clear and helpful comments on the various drafts, for introducing me to the raw lifestyle back in 1994, and for doing what he is doing; Ann Morgan for hosting the Permaculture Course where it all happened back in '94, for being Ann, and to Turners Field for being Turners Field, with its wonderful salads and for the different world that it is; to the people that are Plants for a Future, and all of those involved in PFAF over the years; Elaine Bruce for being such a vibrant example of living foods and permaculture; Sure/Liefde/Kerry Mastin and her many 'cellves' for being light years ahead of the rest of us in creating the extraordinarily real yet different paradise garden reality that Tiaia is, and Aranya for being another living, loving example of the paradise garden way; to all my wonderful friends at Ecoforest, for living their own versions of the Working With Nature way, and helping make Ecoforest happen; Susie Miller for starting FRESH and Karen Knowler for doing so much to take FRESH to the next level; to the US pioneers that are no longer with us such as Arnold Ehret and Ann Wigmore, and to those that are doing it now such as Gabriel Cousens, Douglas Graham and David Klein and others of Healthful Living International, Viktoras Kulvinskus, Paul Nison, David Wolfe and Nature's First Law, Frederic Paténaude and others for their tremendous work around the world; so many authors, teachers and raw food and permaculture activists, past, present and future, all of whom are part of the positive and peaceful (r)evolution towards health and sustainability of which this book is a part; Bill Mollison and David Holmgren for sowing the seeds and doing the 'educational mulching' that started permaculture off, and the permaculture community in the UK, the USA and around the world; to all the raw food pioneers and practitioners, writers and researchers over the years of the 21st and 20th centuries, and before, who have done so much to bring this natural, peaceful way of life and health to so many; all my raw and permaculture friends not mentioned by name for being who you are and doing what you are doing; AND a huge 'thank you' to Maddy, Tim and Patrick Harland, John Adams and the rest of the team at Permanent Publications for their unstintingly positive and supportively critical comments on the various drafts, without which this would not be nearly as effective a package of information and inspiration as people tell me it is. Thank you all.

Steve Charter   **Eat More Raw**

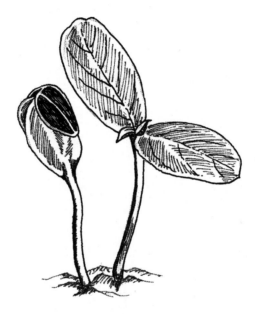

Eat More Raw

Contents

PART TWO
The Practicalities

PART THREE
There Is Plenty of Information And Inspiration Out There

PART FOUR
The Appendices

Foreword

Progress tends to come in spurts. Like the well-known plateaus that people experience in their personal training, all of our learning is subject to periods of hibernation. It takes time to get used to new levels of performance, advances in technology, linguistic nuances, social progress.

Once we get used to the new way and gain some experience in using it, better ways become apparent. Such is growth. That is what this book is all about; bringing the reader to a new found level of awareness.

Specialization is a strong indicator of growth. In the raw food movement, there have been vast waves of specialization in the past few years. Each new aspect of this specialization has raised the awareness of those involved in the movement. It has made it easier for people to succeed as raw fooders, or to better perform their outreach or educational missions. Specialization has helped those already in the movement, but it has not really resulted in growth of the movement. For growth to occur, a bigger overall picture must be observed and put into effect. That, exactly, is what you will find within these pages; a profoundly new perspective that beautifully merges many varied aspects of the healthful lifestyle.

Let me use the sport of golf as an example, for a moment. Golf is an extremely challenging game to play. It is comprised of many aspects. The number of variables are huge. You may get better and better at one aspect of the game but see no indicator of such by an overall lowering of your total end score. Practise as you will, golf can remain extremely frustrating, especially if you are attached to the score as an indicator of how well you played the game.

Then, one day, things come together in a new way. The bits and pieces begin to fall into place. After a few holes, your entire perception of yourself and the game begins to change. A new self confidence arises. You can even express your performance with a vocabulary that until today had eluded you. Lo and behold, at game's end, several strokes have come off of your all time low score. You have evolved.

In much the same way, this book marks the beginning of a new era. It marks the culmination of many years of cultural, environmental, and food style advances. It marks a union of diverse areas of study. Within these pages, what were until now separate and distinct fields of endeavour have come together. They have been artistically united in a fashion that will bring the reader to new found understandings of a bigger picture of healthful living.

We stand on the precipice of survival. We can choose to continue doing what we have always done in the past, in which case the demise of the human race is predictable. We can instead move forward, experiment, and make lifestyle modifications. Armed with better information, humans tend to make better decisions. I believe that reading this book will leave you better informed, make you a better person, and give you many of the tools that you need to emerge from the cultural cocoon as the butterfly that we all wish to become.

Dr Douglas N. Graham (*President of Healthful Living International*)

Introduction

There is a lot more to food than meets the eye...

Our food can be a vehicle for positive personal and planetary change. Alternatively, it can sustain ill-health, economic exploitation and ecological damage. Food and the way we obtain it is connected to a whole network of different effects in our lives and in the world we are part of. Food affects and is affected by activities in the economy, society and the web of life – the outside world. Food is also affected by and affects our internal world – our mind, our body, spirit and emotions.

This book explores and offers guidance on what happens when we eat more raw foods – specifically fresh and organic fruits, vegetables, salads, nuts, seeds, sprouted pulses and grains, cold pressed oils, sea weeds, herbs and so on. It is a book about eating more raw food, whilst also looking at the possibilities of eating only or mainly raw foods. It is about what happens to the chain of effects in your life when you eat more raw foods, and what happens when you grow more of the food you eat. So it's a book that is relevant to you if you eat no raw foods at all; and it's also relevant if you eat 100% raw... and any where in between. It's relevant if you are a meat eater or a vegan, a vegetarian or a chocoholic and junk food addict. It is a book that is relevant if you grow all of your own food... or none of it.

This is a book for people who ask questions about the health of their bodies, the health of their family and friends, and it's also about the health of this rather extraordinary planet we live on; the health of the abundant, varied yet utterly interconnected and evolving eco-systems on which we and all life on the planet depend. It's a book about the effects of what we eat on ourselves and on the world in which we live. So if you care about your home, planet earth, what we are doing now, and how that is affecting the planet, all life on it, your own health and the health of friends, children or relatives then this is a book that you need to read.

This book shows how you can use the food you eat and the cause-and-effect web of relationships that are connected to it to inspire, encourage and accelerate 'Sane, Humane and Ecological' change. In particular this book suggests that by working with nature, it is actually relatively easy to improve the health of people and planet. I hope this book will aid those interested in health, nutrition, organics, permaculture[1] and more ecologically sustainable ways of living.

In particular this book is relevant for people interested in more ethical and ecologically sustainable ways of living, food issues and the relationship between health and nutrition. And it's a book for people that are seeking a

---

[1] Permaculture is a way of creating more ecologically sustainable ways of living, that get more out of life with less hard work; it is defined in more detail on page 39.

1

simple, natural, straight-forward perspective on health and nutrition, that is so different from the technological and drug based view of illness and food that dominates our society in the early 21ˢᵗ century.

If you want to change your life in a positive way, and the inner and outer effects of your life, it is a book for you...

So what's in this book, then? This first part of the book explores and exposes the nature of health and sustainability 'problems' (a negative interpretation) – or if you prefer, health and sustainability 'issues' (which is a neutral interpretation) – or even health and sustainability 'opportunities' (which is the positive interpretation). This first section also details some basic principles that can help you to understand the cause-and-effect nature of the issues, which can then help you to live in more naturally healthy and sustainable ways.

The second and third parts of the book cover the practical 'solutions' to the 'problems'. Or in other words, the positive and creative responses to our situation that will improve our health and increase our sustainability in very straightforward ways. And the fourth part includes some inspirational offerings from wise and experienced friends, with a range of really useful information following in the Appendices... including some delicious raw recipes. Which all sounds pretty good to me, so I hope it does to you too!

Raw Foods - Fad or Feeling?

The main theme of this book is to understand what happens when we eat more raw foods. This idea then naturally extends to understanding what happens when we eat mainly or only raw fruits, vegetables, nuts and seeds, and when we grow more of these foods ourselves. This idea was certainly new to me when was I first told about it! But I listened and then I tried it – and once I tried it I found that in fact it didn't feel strange after all. So let's be clear that whilst it is still unusual to eat mainly or only raw foods, it is not weird at all once one looks into it. The idea may be new to your mind – I found that the reality was and still is that it feels utterly natural to my body!

So is eating more raw foods or eating mainly raw foods (fruit, veg, seed sprouts, nuts, dried fruit, fresh juice, etc.) just for 'nuts'? One of those fads that some people get into? Yes, it certainly is for some people. But emphatically 'No' it is not for the vast majority that try it and continue it. And if you want to know why it's no fad, then all will be revealed within the pages of this book!

In fact eating mainly (i.e. 50% of your diet or more) or only raw foods is highly recommended and seen as essential by a number of notable people. Robert Hart, pioneer of forest gardening in Britain, and an inspiration to so many in the organic, vegan and permaculture movements recommends in his book, *Forest Gardening*, a minimum 70% raw diet for anyone seeking to create a state of positive physical and ecological health. Interestingly, coming from a very different perspective, American success 'guru' Anthony Robbins recommends exactly the same thing in his book *Unlimited Power*, because he sees vibrant health as essential for anyone wanting to be successful in achieving his or her objectives in life.

So people get into raw food for a number of reasons. Some people do try it as a food fad, possibly having tried macrobiotics or the Hay Diet before. Indeed a raw lifestyle is now becoming very fashionable in Hollywood and California, although in many cases famous people, like anyone else, have made this choice for reasons that are far stronger than mere fashion. Some people decide to try eating a lot of raw foods having seen the difference it made to a friend or relation, whilst some may be given or chance upon a book, tape or video that opens their eyes to a whole new world that they had never been aware of before!

In contrast many others find themselves eating a whole lot of raw foods by just following their feelings and intuition, gradually simplifying their diet as they go – listening to their body's natural wisdom. As the body cleanses it becomes easier and easier to hear the body telling you which foods feel really good. This is intuitive eating, which Sibila describes in a later section of this book, and which is also described in more detail in *Feel Good Food* by Susie Miller and Karen Knowler[2].

Others arrive by a path that involves a search for more natural, ethical and sustainable ways of living. Many people feel it is a more compassionate way of life, arriving as a natural extension of vegetarianism or veganism, or being 'green'. Others sense the spiritual benefits, or come to recognise the tradition of eating only or mainly raw fruit amongst gurus in India, or find powerful references in ancient texts, including the *Bhagavad-Gita* and the *Bible*. Some people see that eating mainly raw has clear and numerous ecological benefits as a way of life, whilst many understand its benefits when seeking significantly improved or optimum health and fitness. Within this last group there are some people who are relatively healthy already and who are seeking the healthiest lifestyle they can achieve. And as a perfect example of this, the tennis player Martina Navratilova – probably the most successful sports woman of all time – by becoming 'raw' late in her career she was able to maintain supreme levels of both physical and mental fitness, way after the age at which most athletes start to decline.

Others arrive at raw foods because they have some illness or disease and have heard or read about the important role that a raw food diet can play in enabling healing to take place. Raw foods, particularly green juices and 'living foods' (see Elaine Bruce's section later) have been found by many people to have significant benefits in fighting often frightening 'lifestyle diseases' such as cancer, as well as significantly improving the quality of life of those with arthritis, asthma or eczema. Indeed, I have read that this has brought Muhammad Ali to explore a raw food diet in his ongoing fight against the effects of Parkinson's disease.

[2] Published by The Women's Press, London (2000).

In any situation, the most powerful healing and health creating effects will be felt by adopting a multi-tactic approach, with exercise, meditation, and other significant lifestyle changes – both changing the external conditions that created the disease, and working on the internal conditions to enable healing to take place. Alongside switching to mainly raw foods, meditating and using various therapies, I've heard of people buying a good selection of comedy videos to seriously use laughter in an anti-cancer strategy.

A large number of people explore the raw food lifestyle with an awareness of several of these issues. This fits with the ideas of permaculture – a system of lifestyle and landscape design which always aims to create several benefits from making one key change. (And you'll be pleased to hear that 'the p-word' – permaculture – is described in practical detail later in this book). All this also suggests the simple and appealing idea that we can actually and quite easily eat our way towards health and sustainability!

It is useful to be aware of the social, psychological and emotional pressures against eating mainly raw foods. Food advertising, social norms, and the general lack of open mindedness or health awareness in society all contribute to the challenge and adventure of exploring raw foods. We do know a heck of a lot about illness and disease... and that is simply because western medicine has almost exclusively studied illness and disease – it has not studied health. So, if you look around you today, actually how much do we know about real, positive, natural, vibrant health? How many ordinary people are naturally and vibrantly healthy? What is the 'normal', average state of health, and why? What natural laws determine our state of health? There must be some such natural laws... and knowing nature, they are probably quite simple.

Think for a moment about how much advertising there is for raw fruit and veg – think hard. That's right, virtually none! Meanwhile junk food advertising is everywhere – often with elements of the marketing campaigns directly targeted at kids. Coca Cola is the most well known brand name in the world, with McDonalds not far behind; the ultimate symbols of the civilised, western good life, eh? Which says a lot.

But it's not just the most obviously junky junk foods that are pushed, pushed, pushed at us. There are many cooked food fads for example. And there are the pressures of the heavy sell, addictive, high sugar, and high protein foods – style laden chocolate, ice-creams and coffee ads, and the many and various junk foods. All these can create difficulties for us in our minds and emotions. It's hard enough for us adults, then there are the parents of small children, and those small children themselves – 'gotta catch 'em young if you are to protect and expand your market share you know'. So much so that I have heard that because of all the toys it sells as part of its children's meal packages McDonalds is now evidently classified as the largest 'toy retailer' in the world... I wonder why? If true, this could be considered to be somewhat frightening to many people, given what we know about the effects of fast food on peoples' health. So how come such foods are allowed to be sold whilst at the same time there are moves to control 'natural' medicines? A bizarre state of affairs indeed!

There is a whole range of foods from the worst junk foods, right through to 'health food' snacks, many with far too much sugar and many of the wrong kinds of fats. And all these foods, from the healthy whole foods to the worst kinds of processed junk, all work together supporting the idea that processed and cooked foods in their various forms are perfectly 'normal'. Which means eating a whole lot of raw foods must be a bit 'weird'... perhaps... and then again, perhaps not.

For some people, once they grasp the essence of a more 'natural', more ecological or more intuitive approach to food, all this advertising of 'garbage' food makes it easy to start walking away from (sometimes quite hurriedly!), as they see the craziness of what goes on in our society more vividly. A vital, and relatively easy first step being to walk away from the processed foods that are so obviously unnatural and unhealthy.

Think for a moment about the foods that you know are actually natural foods. Once you look from a fresh and natural perspective it seems pretty clear that most of the very unhealthy foods are usually profitable foods – both for the food producers and sellers, but also for the drug manufacturers, the 'health' industry, the supplement sellers and so on. Meanwhile the most natural foods are naturally the most health creating – it is that simple.

Sickness and the associated fear of ill-health is sold to us as 'normal' and unavoidable, sometimes consciously, sometimes unconsciously, and as a result we have become an increasingly 'junk-food-addicted' and innocently unaware society. All this is a sales hype that can be very easy to walk away from, once you have some choices about where else you can head for.

This can be incredibly liberating. If your health is taken from you then your freedom is certainly reduced, and for many removed completely. Think about that for a moment. Fear of illness greatly reduces our sense of freedom, making us feel we have to have close and immediate access to doctors and hospitals, as well as making us feel we have to keep working away to keep up the medical insurance payments. Once you understand that you can actually take control of your own health then all this can change.

So, eating a lot of raw foods can be a fad for some, but for the majority, a mainly, or totally, raw food lifestyle is the result of a genuine search for an improvement in their lifestyle – either for their own benefit or to benefit their relationship with the planet... and often both of course.

If, when you've read this and possibly other books, you choose to explore eating more raw foods then your lifestyle will change. It will change you and the world around you. In doing so it may be useful to understand that what you are doing is helping to create positive change in your lifestyle; a more positive 'ripple effect'.

Permaculture - Fad or Feeling?

So what about permaculture then? Well, if you want to get a flavour of what permaculture is then you'll find that its central ideas and practices are described later in this book. I will start simply by saying that permaculture has been described as 'probably the most practical of green ideas'. It has also been described as 'applied common sense, in a world where sense is becoming less common'. Permaculture is derived from the idea of establishing a permanent (i.e. sustainable) agriculture and sustainable culture.

One of the biggest problems for those seeking to shift the western, developed nations to a more wise and sustainable path is that the vast majority of people no longer know how to grow food. So they have become trapped and dependent upon industrialised agriculture and the global food market. They therefore have to take what they are given, and lack information as well as quality and true choice, because they lack the choice to grow their own foods, and to meet their wider needs themselves, or with others locally. Permaculture is directly and deliberately designed to help us break out of this trap, and to enable us to enjoy more choice, more freedom and more fulfilment in life, whilst also enabling us to live more responsibly.

A more technical description of permaculture suggests it is about 'designing sustainable lifestyles'. And a definition I have used is that it is about really good observation, and making changes in ourselves and the world around us that are positive and constructive. Its essence is to understand the patterns and the true nature of life, health, sustainability and the world we are part of, and then to work with those patterns and natural processes rather than against them. So permaculture is fundamentally about working with nature, rather than against nature. And it is about designing changes in our lives, and then making those changes, as a route to changing our world. So it's about taking responsibility for our lives.

A number of very useful permaculture tools and techniques are described later in this book, but for the meantime it is enough to know that permaculture is particularly concerned with producing food, whilst also being concerned with how much energy and what type of energy we use, how much waste we produce and what we do with it, where we live and the effects of our general lifestyle. Permaculture is certainly highly adaptable; it's what you make it! And judging by the enthusiastic way in which many people have taken up its ideas it seems that if permaculture is a fad then it is a very useful and enjoyable one.

There is a lot of feeling or 'heart' in the people involved in the permaculture movement, and as with many things, if you really want to know more about that feeling then the best way is to go on a permaculture course, subscribe to *Permaculture Magazine*, visit a local permaculture project or go to a permaculture gathering and find out for yourself (the same goes for raw food courses and gatherings, by the way!).

Why Raw Food and Permaculture?

So why raw food and permaculture? Well, because they go together so well. And the reason they go together so well is that they both work with nature.

Working with nature involves the joyful experience of getting a feel for the web of life and evolution, inside your body and in the world around you – which is ecology. If we are getting a feel for ecology why just look outside the human body? If we really want to understand and practice ecology then we need to look at the ecology of the human body (and mind) as well as the ecology of the environment that the human body is a living, co-existing part of.

What my investigations of permaculture and raw foods have taught me is that ecological sustainability and true, positive health are basically the same types of processes looked at in different contexts – one is about looking at the body, the other is about looking at the world outside, that we are part of. They are both about working with nature.

This book has emerged because it seems logical to me to apply two basic ideas of permaculture to my own 'internal' mind-body-spirit system – firstly that of extended and careful observation, and secondly that of working with nature. So this book is intended to encourage a thoroughly nourishing and wonderfully fruitful exploration of natural, ecological approaches to health and nutrition!

Personally, I do eat mainly raw foods and have done so for many years now (since autumn 1994), and I have had many periods of many months at a time when I've eaten only raw foods, usually mainly fruit with one salad a day. My main intellectual reasons for eating as I do are guided by applying ecological thinking, as well as permaculture ideas and other ethical considerations and principles to my choices of what and how I eat. This is complemented by a healthy dose of well researched information on diet, nutrition and lifestyle –including looking at both what creates sickness, disease and ill-health, and what creates health. And equally importantly, alongside these intellectual reasons, are my intuitive reasons for eating as I do – which are guided by what feels more natural to me, or more accurately what feels good to my body – what 'my body' tells 'me' feels good.

Linking raw food and permaculture is relevant to people all over the world, in virtually all climates. It can be really easy in warm climates where nature makes it easy to grow a wide variety of fruit. In sub-tropical, Mediterranean type and tropical climates, forest gardens, eco-gardens, permaculture systems, organic market gardens and agroforestry can be easily designed to be both beautiful and bountiful; providing many types of vegetables, fruit and herbs all year round that are ideally suited to a high percentage raw diet. They can also provide building materials (timber, bamboo, etc.), fibres, soaps, oils and many other useful plant products.

In a temperate climate (such as Britain and much of northern Europe and North America) the variety is more limited, but is still far, far greater than most people would imagine. A temperate raw food permaculture diet will normally consist fairly equally of salads, leafy greens and fruit, with a range of nuts, seeds and sprouted pulses – a diet that can be very diverse, and much more enjoyable than one might think at first; and certainly much more diverse, more healthy and more sustainable than the typical western diet.

If you want to see change in yourself and changes in the health and sustainability of the world outside, a very important thing to understand is the nature of your own mind and body. And to do that you may need to gain a better understanding of what helps you to understand!

Take a few seconds and think, sense or look into your mind and body to check if you understand things with images in your mind. Alternatively do you understand by getting a bodily feeling or an emotional sense of what feels good or right, or what makes sense? Equally possible is that you understand mainly through words, logic, facts and reason.

Typically each one of us has a dominant mode of understanding; visual (with images in your mind), auditory (through words), or kinesthetic (by feelings and movement).

So, if you really want to help create health and sustainability in your own life and in the world of which you are a part, it will help if you understand what will generate your own understanding of how to do so. Do you need:

a) a set of mental images or a vision of how to create health and sustainability? and/or

b) a feeling, experience or sense of what health and sustainability is? and/or

c) a logical, factual word based understanding that tells you how to create health and sustainability?[3]

If the above seems unnecessary to you don't worry, that's fine; but if it does make sense use it, because it will very probably make a difference!

Without further ado about your mind and you, let's walk on into the garden and see what we find...

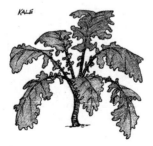

KALE

---

[3] If you want to understand more about how your mind works I strongly recommend *The Mind Map Book* by Tony Buzan (BBC Books) and *From Frogs To Princes* by Bandler and Grinder (Eden Grove Editions, 1990).

Interconnectedness

If you sit in a quiet sunny spot in the garden, or look out at a park or distant hillside, or even just take a really good look at your window box, if you ponder about western science and its theories of relativity, chaos and quantum mechanics, or the spiritual philosophies of Buddhism, Hinduism and Taoism, the Native American traditions, the ancient Egyptian Neters, the mystical aspects of Christianity or the ideas of Epicurus and Heraclietus from Ancient Greece, you will probably find a whole load of differing views of creation that all tell us that all things are interconnected.

Many of the spiritual traditions refer to and draw strongly from nature. Many also refer to the idea of the original paradise as a garden, or an abundant forest.

This universal scientific and spiritual view of life tells us that creation is not something separate, it is here and now, and it is the world we live in day-by-day-by-day... it is us, and we are it... nature, evolution. And they also tell us, both science and the spiritual traditions, that 'reality' differs from our perception of it – and often quite significantly.

We are told from an early age in school about atoms and molecules and so on. We are told that we and everything else, even the clear air around us, is all made up of this 'stuff-that-is-not-stuff', these atoms and molecules. And what's more about 99.9% of those molecules and fundamental particles are nothingness anyway!

So at what point does the oxygen in the air we breathe become part of us? When do the plants we eat stop being part of the environment and become our food? And at what point does the food we eat become part of us? We respond to our environment and our environment responds to us. We shape each other. Where is the division then, if one is part of the other and the 'other' part of one? Is 'nature' outside or in ? Or is it both?

In this sense it is scientifically and spiritually accurate to state that you and your environment are what you eat – the one both creates and is created from the other. However, we are certainly not only what we eat!

Acceptance... or Response-Ability?

Agriculture, industry and the global-to-local economy, as they are now, clearly play a very major role in shaping our environment, both in terms of the landscape that we can see with our eyes, and also in terms of carbon, oxygen and water cycles. And it is our ways of thinking and our values that shape that agriculture, the food industry and the national-global food economy.

The whole food production and supply industry is shaped by what is important to us – in fact generally, it is shaped by what is 'normal' to us. It all reflects the way we think about, or don't think about, our food. It is also a core element in any economy – it cannot be separated from the chemical industry, the energy industry, or from the places that our shops and services hold in our towns. For example, the move towards supermarkets and edge of town shopping, followed by an insidious economic and physical decline and loss of community feeling in many town centres, has been part and parcel of the food industry's never ending drive to cut costs by finding cheaper locations to build cheaper buildings. Supported by our willingness to drive longer distances to avoid town centre congestion, the use of cheaper edge of town sites, the creation of characterless buildings and the employment of many less staff in the food supply chain have all arisen from our desire to make food shopping simple, cheap and convenient – something we just don't have to think too much about in our busy lives.

What happens when we think more about convenience than the quality of the food that we put in our body? The growth of largely 'lifestyle' diseases such as cancer, high blood pressure, stress, tension and illnesses such as ME, all points toward a human metabolism that is generally not very well. Despite the comfort of the modern lifestyle with its cheap and 'convenient' food we are a pretty sick and unhealthy bunch on the whole. How convenient is that for us, our families and friends?

As a society we have masses of information, resources and generally high level of relative affluence, yet large numbers of people make regular visits to the doctor, are continually dropping pills or topping themselves up with a concoction of extra vitamins and minerals.

Do we have to accept all this as it is? What can we do if we do want to change it? Take a few steps back and look at our food system. The way we eat, and what we eat suggests that many things are not quite right. Public warnings about carrots that are overflowing with chemicals and huge sagas about people who ate bits of cattle, which were fed highly processed bits of brain-diseased sheep are symptomatic of something being seriously out of balance. Irradiated food, microwaved food, genetically manipulated food, highly processed, de-natured, junk food... in ignorance of its long term effects, all these are what most people build, maintain and fuel themselves, and their children, with! To me it feels like most of these things should not even be called 'food', let alone good nutrition!

Shouldn't we be asking how this has happened? Could it be because we just don't think much about our food, except in terms of its cost and convenience? These things are produced and supplied as industrial products, not as 'food'.

You can turn things on their head though – and quite simply. Instead of convenience you can place quality and positive reactions in the food chain as top priorities. What is actually most convenient? Having cheap, fresh organic

WHAT'S IN YOUR DRINK? A rough guide...	INSTANT COFFEE or REGULAR TEA	ORGANIC FAIR-TRADE COFFEE or TEA	ORGANIC HERB TEA or COFFEE SUBSTITUTE	FRESH HERBS FROM THE GARDEN
FOOD MILES	MASSIVE	MASSIVE	LESS IF NOT IMPORTED	NONE ☺
ENERGY TO PROCESS & MAKE PRODUCT	HIGH TO VERY HIGH	HIGH TO SIGNIFICANT	HIGH TO SIGNIFICANT	NONE ☺
PACKAGING	PLENTY (too much!)	PLENTY (too much!)	PLENTY (too much!)	NONE ☺
AGRO-CHEMICALS	PLENTY	NONE ☺	NONE ☺	NONE ☺
AGRICULTURAL ENERGY USE	YES	YES	YES	NONE ☺
MULTINATIONAL PROFITS	PLENTY (too much!)	NO ☺	NO ☺	NONE ☺
SUPERMARKET PROFITS	USUALLY (too much!)	DEPENDS ON WHERE YOU BUY IT...	DEPENDS ON WHERE YOU BUY IT...	NONE ☺
ETHICAL ISSUES	IGNORED	CONSIDERED IMPORTANT ☺	POSSIBLY CONSIDERED	NONE ☺
BOILED WATER (ENERGY)	YES	YES	YES	YES BUT CAN BE MADE AS SUN TEA TOO ☺

...AND IF YOU ADD MILK/CREAM OR SUGAR ...YOU CAN DO THE WHOLE EXERCISE AGAIN!

food growing outside your back door, or battling through the aisles and checkout queues piling the trolley high with packets and packages, tins, boxes, bags and bottles? Is it convenient to be afraid of falling sick at any time?

Imagine what happens if we consciously start growing, eating and buying to create positive, healthy lifestyles that create a positive chain of effects in the world. Can you see what a difference this would make? By consuming a higher proportion of food that works with nature you can promote both personal and planetary health, and you can use your consumer power to positively influence the economy too.

As you will see, it can be done and it can be surprisingly easy. On such a path, you will be eating your way to creating significant positive change. What could be simpler?

Personal and Planetary Health

Before we start deciding which path to health and sustainability we should take it makes sense to have a little look around to recognise where we are now in the 'personal and planetary health' landscape.

The WHO (World Health Organisation) definition of health is a 'state of complete mental, physical and social well being and not merely an absence of disease or infirmity'. Based on this definition, and recognising that we are a scientifically and technologically advanced civilisation, what is the norm now for western people? Is it health, as defined by the WHO, or is it some other state of being? And if we are not healthy, what are some of the key causes and effects that deprive us of that complete state of well being?

At the personal level, when it comes to food we are literally the 'consumers' of it, so it makes sense to think about what we are consuming – not just the food itself, but also the chain of effects that got it to your plate... the packaging, the processing, the deals with the suppliers, where it came from originally, the amount of energy, fossil fuels and pollution involved in getting it to you, the kind of landscape or wildlife habitat it creates (or destroys), the philosophy of the company that's selling and marketing it, and so on.

So lets start doing that by looking at some known research on the effects of food on health. Firstly, it is worth noting that an extensive study by the American Medical Association in 1961 showed that vegetarians are dramatically healthier; however, clearly not a great deal has been done to promote this scientifically determined conclusion. In terms of the physical health of the human body there is a huge amount of evidence and experience that shows the numerous benefits of eating a high-percentage-raw diet. Leslie and Susannah Kenton's excellent book *Raw Energy* details many such research studies, including:

※ The work of the Swiss Physician Max Bircher – Brenner in studying the great healing benefits of 'living foods' as he called them.

※ The German physician Max Gerson's work initially on migraine, then on the 'incurable' disease lupus, and most famously on cancer as detailed in his book *A Cancer Therapy: Results of Fifty Cases*.

* The Danish physician Kristine Nolfi's successful personal battle against breast cancer.
* The detailed and rigorous work of the scientist Arnold Ehret looking at fasting and 'the mucousless diet'.
* The extensive work of the American dentist Weston A Price on nutrition and physical degeneration.
* And last but by no means least in this list, the American juice therapy expert Dr Norman Walker (107 and still going strong when *Raw Energy* was published).

More recently we have numerous other experts, including Dr Gabriel Cousens, Dr Douglas Graham, Dr Joel Robbins, Dr Ann Wigmore and the outspoken David Wolfe of the dynamic American organisation Nature's First Law. All these people and many others have studied in great detail what creates and supports health. They have understood that the immune system functions much more effectively when it is fed by a diet that is more natural. And they know that raw plant foods in general are excellent sources of all the nutrients we need for vital and vibrant health, and that some particular foods have specific beneficial effects. David Wolfe points out that if you want to be successful in creating excellent health you have to seek out and study those that are supremely healthy.

Alongside the information that modern science provides on such foods, many spiritual traditions also recognise the benefits of raw food eating and/or fasting. So this knowledge is not new; it has been around for thousands of years. But it has seemed a little hidden until recently – perhaps because it is less profitable and leads to less dependence on drugs and well paid experts. It is certainly not new – it is tried, tested and proven. Its positive effects can and have been observed and repeated again and again.

It's also well worth considering research into the successes and effects of conventional medicine, as well as research into the life expectancy of humans around the world. An American doctor who has carried out extensive research in this area is Dr Joel Wallach, who recorded a fascinating talk entitled 'Dead Doctors Don't Lie' in July 1994. In this talk Dr Wallach, who was a specialist vet before he went on to train as a doctor, discusses a research project he was involved in during which he carried out around 17,500 autopsies on 454 species of animals, and around 3,000 autopsies on human beings. His conclusions from this research were that every animal and every human being that dies of 'natural causes' dies because of a nutritional deficiency.

Dr Wallach emphasises that the scientifically accepted view is that the genetic potential for longevity of human beings suggests we should live to around 120 to 140 years old. Clearly this is not the norm... However, it is also not necessarily as unusual as we might think. Dr Wallach lists a few cases to indicate this: the Hunza Indians of East Pakistan who are relatively well known for living to 120 to 140 years, Russian Georgians who commonly live to 120, and the Armenians and Ebkanians, where living to 120 or 140 is not uncommon. He cites one Armenian who, from his military records, is thought to have lived to 167 years old. Then in South America there's the Vilcabamba Indians of the Ecuadorian Andes and the Titicaca Indians of south east Peru who regularly have lived to 120 to 140 years old. Switching continents he then cites the case of a chief in Niger who died at 126 years old with all his teeth, and a Syrian gentleman who is in the *Guinness Book of Records*... because he fathered 9 children after he was 80 years old and went on to live to 133.

Interesting figures perhaps, but so what? Perhaps more significant is that in 1994 the average age at death in the USA was 75.5 years old. Whilst, American doctors on average died at the age of 58... which says a lot. Dr Wallach states that these figures suggest there is a great value in treating yourself, rather than putting your health in the hands of doctors.

As a result of his research Dr Wallach practiced for many years using nutrition with his patients, pointing out that if they followed his advice properly they were certain to add many healthy years to their life, as well as 'saving a gob of money' in the process. He went much further too. In the talk he quotes a 3 year study by the well known consumer activist Ralph Nader, published in 1993 on the causes of death in US hospitals. Quoting this study he states that '300,000 Americans are killed each year in hospitals alone as a result of medical negligence'. He puts this shocking statistic in context by pointing out that in the 10 years of the Vietnam war US military losses were around 56,000, leading to vast protests and demonstrations. Yet, according to the Nader study around five times that many people were 'being killed' each year inside America's own hospitals by medical negligence... without any mass protest at all. Why?

Let's briefly look at the norms again:
How things are now...

In the UK 1 in 12 women develop breast cancer – 80% of them having no family history of the disease...
Look at trends in sterility and couples' ability to have children – about 1 in 4 couples in Britain are having difficulty conceiving.
The USA has the highest incidence of osteoporosis in the world.
Virtually no one in the western world dies a natural, healthy death of 'old age' – the vast majority die of degenerative lifestyle diseases, in particular cancer and heart disease.

It is worth noting that whilst higher incomes in general lead to longer life expectancy it is also the case that wealth does not equal health. Hugely wealthy industrialists, such as Sir James Goldsmith, die of heart disease and cancer in their 50s and 60s just like the rest. They can pay to be kept alive longer in their very unhealthy state because they can afford the very best treatment for the very worst states of health. But their wealth does not make them healthy. Whilst health care insurance and treatment for ill-health may be expensive, health itself is not. Health can be achieved on a very low income, a middle income or a high income – true, natural, vibrant health does not discriminate, as can be seen from Dr Wallach's studies of the tribes and people that live longest.

So what is the point to all these figures and statistics? The point is to question what is really happening with our health. And with your health. The point is to ask: what makes the difference between health and longevity, and sickness, disease and an early death? And the point is to ask: is it a simple or complex difference? Look out for 'Pottenger's Cats' later in the book and you may find out...

A Healthy or Unhealthy Future?

Health is a key factor in people's quality of life – and a sustainable society implies a healthy society. So how is western society doing in meeting our need for health? An extremely informative and entertaining taped lecture by Dr Joel Robbins' called *Health Through Nutrition* describes America's depth of understanding when it comes to health creation[4]. It indicates the nature of US society whilst also painting a picture that reflects western society in general – where America leads the rest often follow. Early in his talk Dr Robbins states some fascinating facts:

"In 1900, of people over 40 years old, 20 per cent suffered from one or more chronic degenerative diseases – that's cancer, arthritis, diabetes, heart disease and so on.

Since 1900 we have gained more knowledge in the area of health and disease than in all of history combined. We have more medical research per capita than any nation, and more money going into medicine than any nation. The hospital industry is the fifth largest industry in the USA. We have the best doctor : patient ratio of any nation in the world.

Let's go back to that original statistic. In 1900, 20 per cent of people over 40 suffered from some chronic degenerative disease. With all the medical advances we have acquired since 1900, what do you think has happened to that percentage? It's got to have gone down right? We're smarter, we know more about how this body works, we have better medication, right?

Today, 70 per cent of people over 40 suffer from a chronic degenerative disease. That doesn't make sense. It doesn't make sense at all."

That extract tells us so much. It might be useful to read it again because it suggests we are facing a longer-lived but at the same time an increasingly unhealthy future. Which means massive amounts of disease related pain and suffering, and huge and rising health costs, as well as huge profits for the drug and medical industry, the industries that need high levels of sickness, ill-health and disease to be profitable. Based on their current approaches government, the 'health'/drug industry and the medical professions will not reverse this

---

[4]   Dr Joel Robbins, *Health Through Nutrition*, Health Dynamics Corp., 6711 South Yale, Suite 106, Tulsa, Oklahoma 74136. Tel: 1 800 653 5444 in USA.

because, as Dr Robbins' quote points out, they already know more than ever before about illness and already spend more than ever before on health... yet still we are getting sicker, even though we are also living longer in ill-health because of these drugs.

But what if there was a relatively simple answer to health? What if it was staring us in the face, but because it was so obvious we failed to see it? What if we could live longer and be healthy too?

One of Dr Robbins' main points is that given half a chance nature naturally creates health – it is that simple. But, at the same time the first priority is survival. True health can only emerge if the body is not using up most of its energy trying to survive. And most of us are throwing so much processed and junk food into our bodies, living highly stressful lives, in a polluted environment that a lot of our energy just goes into survival. We have no energy or resources left to create or maintain health, so gradually as we grow older we grow sicker and sicker – or as often happens, we go over a threshold level and suddenly discover we are very sick, the disease having been hidden by the body's ability to survive. Think how many people suddenly discover they have serious cancer.

If we are creating so much illness, we are clearly not working with nature. We are not giving our bodies the chance to create health, because the body is constantly battling to survive against illness, stress and pollution. To use Dr Robbins' phrase we are not working with the body's 'innate intelligence'.

We do know how to keep people alive longer, to survive for longer – and this is clearly positive. However, lifestyle diseases are proliferating – cancers, ME and heart disease are some examples, and diabetes is another now common mainly western 'disease' along with asthma. We probably all have friends or relatives who have suffered from one or more of these distressing and expensive conditions. Although medical knowledge is keeping us alive longer, more people are suffering from degenerative diseases and/or are unhealthy and obese, and at a younger age. Sickness is thriving because, generally, the way we choose to live makes us increasingly sick and unhealthy.

With a natural understanding of health this absence of wellbeing can be explained, and we can choose to change the situation. For example, a growing concern for parents of young babies is known as 'Failure to Thrive'. From the conventional point of view Failure to Thrive (FTT) has been largely unexplained. On the other hand, from a perspective that understands the natural nature of health it is easy to identify reasons for its growth. We are no different to other living systems in that we thrive if we have our basic needs met, as nature intends. Therefore, Failure to Thrive is the natural and inevitable product of our failure to supply the natural needs of our body/mind system for ourselves and our children. As a natural result FTT emerges, because unknowingly the parents' bodies are unable to provide the full natural needs to the baby, before and after it is born. This is a failure to work with nature.

In the UK Professor Robert Winston, the well known expert in human reproduction, advisor to the UK government and regular presenter of TV programmes on health and the human body, is now making it clear that the long term health of each and every human being is directly linked to the quality of nutrition that the mother eats during pregnancy.

The 'crisp culture', the culture of the deep freeze, the microwave and junk food has really only taken off since the 1970s. Because of the incredible adaptability and resilience of our bodies, particularly when young, the long term side effects of such a highly processed diet take time to emerge. What's more since the '60s there have also been:

* Massive increases in commercial and industrial chemical use, particularly chlorine chemistry, toxic waste, etc.

* Massive increases in the use of pesticides, artificial fertilisers, growth hormones and other agro-chemicals.

* Rising levels of urban air pollution, particularly associated with traffic growth in the 1980s.

We have never ever had a generation before this time that has grown up and started to produce the next generation, having lived all their life eating and surrounded by this sort of stuff – which in nutritional terms we could term 'absolute garbage'. Which means adult bodies (including their eggs and sperm) built out of nutritional 'garbage'. So we are talking about a living system (the human body and mind) having more and more toxins fed into it, with a static or weakening capacity to tackle those toxins[5].

Pottenger's Cats - an Omen for the Junk Food Lifestyle?

The 'Pottenger's Cats' experiments[6] from way back before the Second World War have daunting implications for a junk food culture. These experiments by the American physician Dr Francis M Pottenger involved feeding around 800 cats a diet of meat, milk and cod liver oil, one group with raw meat (i.e. natural) and the other with cooked meat (i.e. processed). The detailed research found that it took three generations for the full effects of the difference in diet to come through, with noticeable effects in the second generation.

Amongst the cats fed on the highly processed food, the second generation started developing serious degenerative diseases in their middle age. The third generation started seeing degenerative diseases emerging from birth. And as for the fourth generation? There was no fourth generation. The third generation was either sterile or aborted the foetus... no fourth generation.

Now think about the current trends in human health and fertility in the west.

---

[5] Technically speaking a 'toxin' is a substance that takes energy to process and get out of the body, and which provides little or no nutritional value. It is a drain on the system. The more extreme the toxin the more energy is needed to get it out of the body, therefore the more it depletes the body's energy and resources.

[6] I do not endorse animal experimention at all. I quote the Pottenger's Cats experiment on the basis that I do not consider the lives of those cats as worthless, or wish them to be forgotten.

It would be foolish to directly compare humans and cats, as clearly humans are more adaptable in their diet. However, with the growth of lifestyle diseases, falling fertility and the predominance of the microwaved, packaged, processed, junk food culture, it would probably be far more foolish to dismiss or ignore the lessons of Pottenger's Cats because they are clearly extremely relevant to an early 21st century human diet that is full of highly processed food. Just think of all those highly processed factory foods that most of us eat without a second thought.

With an understanding of nature we can explain why Dr Francis Pottenger found what he did. Nature designed neither cats nor humans to eat processed food – or to live in a highly toxic and stressful environment. The basic drive in nature is to survive and reproduce – survival comes first, health only comes if there is enough energy left. The body, 'assumes' that it will be fed naturally. But when faced with the 'processed food and toxic environment' situation the pattern is that the body manages to survive, but it has no energy or resources left to create health.

The pattern in nature is that when it has a choice about a pregnant mother, nature normally prioritises the survival of the mother – because the mother has survived the most vulnerable years of life and is already at breeding age. But the mother won't be healthy if she's eating unhealthy foods. So her unhealthy body just cannot build a healthier foetus than the nutrition it is provided with allows. This is why when we eat an unnatural, highly processed diet each generation gets a worse start than its parents did. The foetus is likely to be built out of more toxic and poorer quality materials than the mother, every time. So illness, unhealthiness and disease show up earlier and earlier in each generation's life; the children get sicker sooner, and the grandchildren sooner still, possibly from birth.

It is hard enough knowing these facts. It can be harder still for the innocent and unknowing parents and children. These are hard facts to face, especially for mothers that are reading them, and for fathers too. But surely we have to face these facts if we are to move forward to something better that will create less suffering for parents and children, relatives, partners and friends.

But it's not just about food. Pollution, stress and general lifestyle all play their role in the big picture of personal and planetary health and ill-health. But perhaps it is most obvious where food is concerned. Until the 1950's virtually all food was basically organic and far less processed. Almost everywhere I go I now see children and teenagers eating junk food, as well as toddlers in pushchairs being given crisps, canned drinks and junk food snacks full of sugar and additives. It was not like this when I was a kid 30 years ago. Remember, I've been told that McDonalds can be categorised as the biggest toy retailer in the world now... is it selling real health, real quality and real choice with those take-away toys?

The evidence from research suggests that by the time the first chemicalised, junk food generation of humans reach their 30s and 40s the effects will start to show through very clearly in their own health – and the effects will be even clearer in their children. I find this a sad and horrifyingly unnecessary vision for the future.

At this point, please remember that we can all learn to work with nature. The solutions are natural and healthy – and they taste good! The body's innate intelligence is still in good shape, but it does need good quality materials if it is to build a healthy body and mind. An important extra fact from the Pottenger's experiment is that once the third generation cats were switched back to raw foods it took just four generations to achieve full, vibrant health.

The more of us there are eating more organic raw health creating foods, the more quickly the ripple effects of positive health will naturally swell and flow through society. Just look at how the movement against GMOs grew so quickly in the UK.

There are many examples of our poor knowledge of basic nutrition, biology and chemistry. For example, if milk is supposed to provide us with calcium, how is it that Americans, who consume more dairy produce than any other nation in the world, also have the highest rates of calcium deficiency?[7] The answer is that pasteurising milk kills the enzymes needed to digest it properly. This means that the calcium in milk is no longer organically bound and digestible. Our body cannot properly assimilate this inorganic calcium, so it tries to get rid of it where it can, and when it can't flush it through (because of the mucus that dairy and wheat products create in our bodies) it deposits the inorganic calcium where it can in the body – which often means in the joints, thus causing osteo-arthritis. So despite the marketing myths, because the body cannot properly assimilate the inorganic calcium, milk does nothing to prevent osteoporosis (loss of bone calcium), a disease which it is now considered 'normal' for mature Americans!

Even the simplest ideas in living nutrition are generally hidden from us. For example, we just cannot properly digest our food without the full complement of minerals, vitamins and enzymes in our food – they all need to work together for proper digestion. You can't fully take advantage of the minerals and vitamins unless the enzymes are there too.

Enzymes are vital in being able to turn food into nutrition – in other words to digest the food we put into our body. They are intimately linked with life itself, and we have to employ the services of enzymes to break down what we put into our body. There are three types of enzymes: food enzymes, digestive enzymes and bodily enzymes. The food enzymes come into our body in living, raw foods and are the most efficient and ideally suited enzymes to break down that food. Digestive enzymes exist in our digestive system and are the second most efficient type of enzymes for breaking down food. Bodily enzymes are the least efficient for digestion, having to be drawn from other functions to do a job they were not designed for.

7   Joel Robbins, *Health Through Nutrition*.

If we are using digestive enzymes or bodily enzymes they have to be replenished, which draws on our energy and other bodily resources.

When heated to above about 120°F/42°C the vital, living enzymes that are contained in raw vegetables and fruit, and which are needed for proper digestion, are killed – so in effect the food becomes dead. Food moves from biology to chemistry. What this means is that we are constantly putting food in our body which is unnatural, or 'de-natured' (i.e. cooked and processed foods), and which therefore requires our body to manufacture enzymes. In this way we are constantly draining the body of its life force, leading to physical degeneration, illness, disease and premature ageing. Whereas if we put whole, raw, organic plant foods in our body, we are constantly replenishing the body's life force.

So we put biologically inactive, 'dead' food in our body. What other creature on earth does this?

Even veggie burgers and so called 'health foods' take their toll. Most supplements that are pedalled by the chain 'health' stores are expensive and of dubious benefit because they don't have the living enzymes in them that enable us to assimilate them in their inorganic form. Perhaps they are better than nothing – but they are certainly nowhere near as good as getting the vitamins and minerals in their natural packages – fruit and vegetables, which are also far cheaper with far less packaging, processing and promotion.

What we eat is what builds and fuels our minds and bodies – or it gradually demolishes them.

Which would you prefer having your mind and body built out of?

a) greasy and stodgy dead 'food'? or

b) vibrant, crisp and fresh fruit, herbs and vegetables?

If your brain and body is being built of burgers, coke and crisps how will you feel in five, ten or thirty years time? Imagine the differences in your body these diets will create – compare your picture of yourself with a junk food body with your picture of a vibrant, 'raw' body.

Look around yourself at the average state of health of someone 10, 20 or 30 years older than you. They probably got a better start than you. Do you want that state of health for yourself in 10, 20 or 30 years time? Or do you want to do something to create much better health for yourself, and perhaps your children too?

Our food, our bodies, and the bodies of our children are bio-chemical cocktails. Logically it is pretty obvious that our mind-body-spirit is significantly affected by the particular bio-chemical food mixtures that we add into our mind-body-spirit cocktail.

But you are not just your body – you are a mind and consciousness embodied in a body! And because the body is a constant flow of foods, air and liquids, logical reasoning suggests that you/your consciousness is greatly affected by what you eat, i.e. the materials that your consciousness is housed in and fuelled by. So both intuitively and logically it is clear to me that the 'food' that builds, maintains and fuels us is a major factor affecting the overall health and functioning of our whole mind-body-spirit; including our mind and consciousness. I do not mean that just eating raw food will sort out our mind and consciousness and make it pure and brilliant and clean. What I mean is that over the generations, humans have been eating non-evolutionary, inappropriate foods which must have had an effect on the physical-biological quality of our neurosystems, which are our consciousness-generating system. If there has been an effect there is no question that it would have been intensified significantly during the last thirty to fifty years during which the worst of the highly unnatural processed foods have emerged. If a machine is built out of unsuitable materials it just cannot function properly. And this has to be the case even if it is a delicate living, thinking machine, which thinks its limited experience of food and life is 'normal'.

Could it just possibly be the case that the food we use to build, maintain and fuel our mind-body-spirit system has a significant (though not total) effect on the most complex, delicate and sophisticated aspects of our body's neurological system? Which is also the most sophisticated and delicate biological system we know of in all creation. Could it be that because it is no longer built out of natural foods it finds difficulty in recognising those natural foods?

We know foods affect testosterone and other hormone levels, and that these chemicals have a very powerful effect on our behaviour and thinking[8], as well as a huge and critical effect on our growth and development. If our hormones, and our natural steroid balance in particular is out of balance it has to have an effect on our growth and development. It is impossible for it not to have an effect as steroids are the growth regulators that switch on the genes. If you change the steroid balance you get a different genetic outcome. It is that simple – and it definitely warrants further investigation, particularly since high testosterone levels have been found to inhibit neural development in children. If our testosterone levels are higher than nature intended, and we are not getting the neural growth that nature intended, then we are just not getting the brain, neurosystem and body that we are programmed to have in our genes.[9] If this is the case, then this situation could be turned around over two, three or four generations if we get the balance right.

Personally I feel that the state of the world and humanity directly reflects the state of human consciousness – and this is an issue that demands attention if we are wise. It is not something to hide away from. If the current

[8] This is backed up by the research of the Behavioural Health Partnership and many others.

[9] If these issues interest you particularly then visit the website for Experimental Consciousness Research at http://web.ukonline.co.uk/ecr/ also look out for a book by Tony Wright of potentially huge significance, that should be published soon.

state of the world reflects a 'crisis' then what role does food and a toxic environment play in this?[10] Our food is not responsible for it all, but it must play some significant part. And what role might more optimum foods for our mind, body and spirit play in a positive, creative response to the health and sustainability crisis, the major effects of which are only now starting to emerge?

You'll be pleased to hear that there are some answers to such questions in later sections of this book. To polish off this section first though, it makes sense to briefly consider the role our economy plays in creating and maintaining our current food situation; to recognise how our economy also reflects our state of consciousness; and to consider how your role as a 'consumer' supports or changes the economy.

A Healthy Economy?

How does physical health relate to economic health? According to economic theory, an economy is a system for distributing resources, goods and services to meet human needs. So theoretically a healthy economy should be a system that is efficient and effective in meeting human needs.

So what are our needs? There are the obvious physical needs for good food and shelter. Also there are needs for fulfilment that in theory are provided through education, employment, artistic, creative and sporting activities. Then there are the kind of needs that are spoken of in the American constitution – life, liberty and the pursuit of happiness, alongside the need for love and companionship.

Certainly a healthy, modern economy should be involved in making sure that the most important of these needs are being met. I would also suggest that a healthy, intelligent and sustainable economy, in a wise society, should obviously be a health-creating economy, since health is a basic need and a key factor in quality of life. Do we have a health-creating economy? Clearly not if we consider Joel Robbins' facts again. Why?

Part of the reason is that somewhere along the line, probably near its beginnings, economic theory became disconnected from reality, even though it believed and still believes it reflects reality. Related to this, political priorities have become weirdly but understandably distorted so that they are dominated by a limited and limiting range of economic priorities.

Doing something as sensible as actually creating health doesn't fit easily into that puzzle of economic and political priorities. And we don't understand how to create health anyway as our patterns of thinking have lead to distorted pathways of research and therefore a distorted understanding of what constitutes 'good' food and nutrition. So spending more and more money on the increasingly and innocently sick society becomes the priority instead,

[10] I do not feel that just by changing what we eat a 'crisis of consciousness' can be solved – the issues are a little more complex than that! But I know that food is both a central part of the problem... and of the solutions.

because it is assumed that being as sick as this is 'normal' for humans – even for humans in a 'civilised', intelligent and 'developed' society that is quite capable of working out and learning how to live healthily and sustainably... but which isn't doing it!

Another part of the reason why we do not have a health-creating economy is that businesses respond to 'demand' – and demand is what people 'want' to buy(or think they want to buy)and have the money to buy. The problem is that people in a modern western economy can generally only buy what companies have to sell. And very few companies are selling real health (although they will sell you as many so called 'health products' as you wish to buy) because you do not need to buy any products from any company to create health! So raw food nutrition and ecological growing systems are massively liberating, if you want to free yourself from the corporate, all consuming world.

As Dr Joel Wallach points out, being a medical doctor in the US can be a very successful way to earn a great deal of money. He points out that in the USA a heart by-pass operation costs around $100,000, and a great many doctors drive Mercedes. In China doctors traditionally got paid according to how healthy their patients were, not how sick they were.

Business and industry exist to make a profit for their owners – that is their primary purpose. I am not saying that is 'good' or 'bad'; I am saying that's how it is. So the priority for agricultural, food and medical businesses is to survive and make a 'healthy' (sic?) profit – creating health is not a priority. Currently it is more profitable to supply foods that create illness, which then creates profitable business. That is just how it is. All the processing and packaging of foods is done for economic reasons, not health reasons. But... this does not mean we cannot find much healthier and equally economic ways of living and eating... The WTO, G8, businesses and government 'health' services will not do it for us though. That is just how it is.

We need to make a significant shift in ourselves as individual consumers, families and communities. We need to take responsibility for our health and for changing patterns of agriculture and land-use by changing what we eat and how we obtain what we eat. This is the most practical, cheap, effective and democratic policy for health creation. And it is the best and most direct route to a health-creating economy.

A living, positive, creative philosophy of compassion for life, the planet, myself and other humans feels good to me as a way of taking responsibility for my own existence. I am not saying you will be a 'better' person if you do this or that; and I am not telling you to do this or that – that is your decision. What I am aiming for is to provide information and broaden the choices that you have available in taking responsibility for your own existence.

The Prime Directive of Permaculture, According to Bill Mollison:[11]
The only ethical decision is to take responsibility for our own existence and that of our children. Make it now.

Accepting what we are given is no good if we want change. We have to respond positively to shift the margins. The reality is that economies and businesses do respond to demand – because they live and die according to their 'marginal' costs and profits (i.e. a small percentage change in income or costs often makes a big difference to businesses profits – and if profits do fall then businesses change what they are doing, and/or the Chief Executive gets fired). What this means is that if 'we', as only a small percentage of the total market, shift our purchasing patterns then we shift the margins and significantly affect the market as a whole.

Think about the implications, the inter-connected links in the chain; sense the opportunities – a healthy and peaceful apple and salad based revolution perhaps! Russets and rocket salad lead the way! And don't worry about jobs and economic health; these follow demand so we just need to create a healthy demand for all the useful, health creating and positive work that quite obviously needs doing.

If I was to help set up The Health and Sustainability Party, I would feel very comfortable making the following Manifesto commitment:

I hereby guarantee that there will be significant long term reductions in the demands upon and the costs of running the health service for any government or health authority that integrates into its health strategy and rigorously pursues targets for the majority of the population to eat at least 25% of their fruit and vegetables raw, and a further significant proportion of the population to be eating at least 50% of their diet as raw fruits and vegetables.

It might take a while, but if, as a start, 2% or 5% of us ate 90% raw or more, and 10% to 20% ate 50% raw with a high proportion of fruit, that would significantly change the market, and it would improve many people's health. If half of all vegetarians and vegans, and half of all the environmental activists and conscious consumers aimed to eat at least 50% raw for one year we would see the effects. And the effects would definitely be noticeable, significant and very, very positive – for people and planet. For a start it would lead to many more fruit trees being planted, to meet the rising demand for fruit – and trees are much better for the planet than mono-cultural wheat and arable deserts... If you are a vegetarian or vegan, an environmental activist or a conscious consumer I hope you can feel how this simple action might fit well with the ethics and actions you have chosen in your life.

---

[11] Quoted right at the start of *Permaculture: A Designers' Manual* (Tagari Press), the 'Bible' of permaculture written by Bill Mollison.

Health and Sustainability: Where Are We Going?

When we pull together the current trends around us we see:

* Greater ill-health and illness; more people able to survive in a fundamentally unhealthy state.
* Rising global economic centralisation and uncertainty.
* High levels of crime and higher levels of fear of crime.
* An almost complete lack of confidence in our health and therefore in our future, with widespread certainty and acceptance of unhealthiness and disease.
* The illegal drugs trade is one of the biggest industries around the world, especially in the most 'developed' and 'civilised' societies.
* The legal drugs and pharmaceutical trade is another of the biggest industries around the world.
* The break down of communities and a growing 'fortress culture'.
* General disillusionment with the system, politics and the media.
* Environmental degradation, global desertification and gradual climate change.

It's not all bad though! Achieving health and sustainability depends on how we collect and use the information and knowledge at our disposal. Information is a product of learning and we have never had more information available. Wisdom, however, depends on how we use that information. What I see is that our society is over-loaded with information, whilst at the same time having a distinct lack of wisdom. In the sea of information, we are often drowning in quantity, with quality becoming more and more diluted.

Learning implies changes in the way we do things – it is not just an accumulation of facts. Learning is dependent upon our thinking and values motivating us to change our lifestyle. Learning also implies that we know we have something to learn – intellectual humbleness as opposed to intellectual arrogance or naivety. And when it comes to sustainability and health, the wise know that nature is our best teacher – and ultimately is our only teacher.

In western societies we are dominated by technology – when we do learn from nature there is almost always another human being, a computer or a book in between us and nature. We often seek new prophets or gurus to provide us with the ultimate solution to our happiness. We don't realise that it is the vehicle that we are travelling in that provides the lessons.

You are nature, embodied in human form. Through our continual interaction with life, the universe and everything we are all plugged into nature and evolution. We are the universe looking at itself; consciousness embodied in the human body is the universe and nature attempting to understand itself and consciously interact with itself. Are we yet conscious of and making the most of that fact?

Where do you see us heading? Do you want to join others and change direction to a different path with more hope of taking us towards a healthy, sustainable and fulfilling culture?

Whole Health

The picture of health and sustainability can change, but only if we do the painting of it ourselves. If we are to develop any kind of wholeness in health we will need a package that creates health in mind, body, spirit and emotions. This may need us to rewrite our traditional mental stories about ourselves and our society, and to change our goals. This might include:

* At least 50% raw, life-giving, health creating foods, with intelligent use of knowledge of their benefits and effects.
* Meditation, massage and other stress relief or relaxation techniques.
* Exercise and good breathing – yoga, tai chi, the Five Tibetans, etc.
* Clean, fresh air and water.
* Support groups such as co-counselling.
* A range of physical and emotional therapies.
* Artistic and creative activities.
* Some kind of spiritual openness to growth and exploration.
* Plenty of opportunities for contact with nature, plants and the soil.
* Community for shared child care, friendship and diversity, enabling relationships that are not constrained by the typical nuclear family set-up – a move to more diverse, natural and sustainable extended community-families.

With such a package of health creating activities, a revolution in personal and planetary health will naturally result, and the illness and dependency of conventional consumer society will evolve to something more positive, more healthy and more sustainable. All you have to do is sense how to set the creative, healthy forces of nature free in your life as a whole, and in its various elements that make up the whole. And then take the practical, achievable steps to make it happen.

If anyone thinks this is unrealistic, then sit down and take a really long hard look at the current trends in health and healthcare costs, or rather sickness-care costs...

Life in the 21st Century... So What Now?

What are the practicalities of where we are now? As a society where are we heading? Where do we want to be?

Half the world's river water is being used to irrigate crops. Potatoes are most efficient in agro-industry terms – they need 500 litres/kg, chickens need 3,500 litres/kg, and beef requires 100,000 litres/kg.

In East Anglia (UK) for every 1 ton of wheat harvested about 5 tons of soil is lost. At least 80% of arable land in Britain is used to grow fodder for animals.

Australia has the highest incidence of cancer in the world – and is the world's largest red meat consumer. The US eats more food and dairy produce than any other nation – 70% of Americans over 40 suffer from some degenerative disease and the US has the highest incidence of calcium deficiency in the world.[12]

Looking at things in very simple terms, we know that a typical western life expectancy is somewhere between 50 and 80 years. Scientifically it is accepted that the human body is designed to live to around 120 to 130 years. And research into the longest lived tribes on the planet confirms this, showing that it can be common place, and that people can live healthily and actively to this ripe old age, dying without great pain or suffering. What this means is that something in the western lifestyle is denying virtually everyone, including you, virtually half of your life. Something is killing you, and before that putting you in a sad state of health and dependence on support, 40, 50 or 60 years before you are meant to die.

Conventional agriculture relies on highly unnatural plants that have been manipulated to produce strains with a very high starch/sugar content. Through these manipulations the plants become very weak and severely depleted in their mineral content. So, whilst agriculture produces huge volumes of 'food' it does far more to deny us good nutrition than it does to provide it. We can change this. And we can gain the excellent nutrition and health that we all deserve as human beings if we really start to think carefully, and start to consciously design our food growing systems and our diets to provide ourselves with the nutrition that will naturally and automatically create health.

Imagine how all those statistics above would change if 25% or 50% of what we ate was whole organic fruit from trees – made up of the many more varieties and flavours of apples, avocados, apricots, pears, oranges, mangos, grapes, melons and so on than we are currently offered. Imagine what would happen if half the population grew its own vibrant, organic, mineral rich perennial green leafy salads, freshly picked from the garden every day. How would this change water demand, chemical use and soil loss? How would it affect our health? How would it affect your life and your health if you made these changes in your life? How might those changes then positively affect others around you?

Human health and sustainability are totally dependent on our own species' ability and willingness to learn. We know our current path is *not* achieving health or sustainability, so we still have a lot to learn. The information is here with us now, we just have to use it more wisely.

Something major has to shift if we are to break the unhealthy and fundamentally unsustainable continuum. To change the strange loop, at some point we have to step in and make decisions – we have to make a firm choice and take responsibility for changing ourselves.

That's enough about the problems; let's use the nature of the problem to understand and implement 'solutions' – positive, conscious, creative responses that work with nature. Yeeehaaa – here we go...

---

[12] Sources: *Sustainable Somerset New Digest 28*; Permaculture Introductory Course with Phil Corbett, Leicester, Spring 1994; Dr Joel Robbins tape, *Health Through Nutrition*.

A Philosophy Of, And For, Life

The principle of working with nature is highly applicable to diet – in considering both how our diet influences our own natural mind-body-spirit system, and the implications for our immediate environment, the local community, society as a whole, the economy and the wider environment.

To work with nature, not against it is one of the basic principles of permaculture. Even on its own, the principle of working with nature is utterly practical and it provides the foundations for a sane, humane and ecological, as well as healthy and sustainable philosophy for life.

As you may have gathered by now, I feel deep concern about the state of the world. And at the same time I see the awesome creative potential of humanity. So much of that potential appears to be wasted, squashed or misdirected. So I really believe that we can and should be creating something better for ourselves and for our children and grandchildren. And I realise that many people think they are doing this in prioritising economic growth above all else. But in its present form it just is not a sustainable and evolutionary path for humanity[13]. So if we really do want to pursue a positive sustainable path, either we need to change the nature and form of economic development and our economic priorities, or we have to change our other individual and social priorities – or do both of course.

Let's just take a brief look at what 'evolution' is. To me evolution means a significant development in our nature. Given the situation we are in at present, for humanity I feel this means a shift to 'conscious evolution', and this means consciously working with nature – I don't necessarily mean evolution in the Darwinian sense. This means using the vast amounts of information we have available more consciously and much more wisely[14]. It means becoming more aware of the unique nature of our bodies as living systems, our consciousness, our patterns of understanding and misunderstanding, and our patterns of choices – what we choose to do and what we consciously or unconsciously choose to run away from or resist.

It also means working with nature in a far more sophisticated way. This needs us to create a time where we understand nature and evolution to such an extent that it becomes obvious that the most positive path is to work with our own nature, our own consciousness and our own evolution, within the context of the wider nature and evolution of which we are a part. To do that we need to create a positive vision of where we want to be in the future, as well as a practical vision of what steps we need to take now to start us on that path.

---

[13] For more information on sustainability and sustainable development, their background general principles, their economic, social and environmental aspects, as well as its relationship to consciousness, the history of human development and culture, and their relationship to the individual see *The Earth Dweller's Guide to Sustainability*, also by Steve Charter.

[14] For example this would lead to a natural evolution of 'Information Technology' into 'Wisdom Technology' – anyone who wants to take hold of this idea and develop genuine wisdom technology is free to do so!

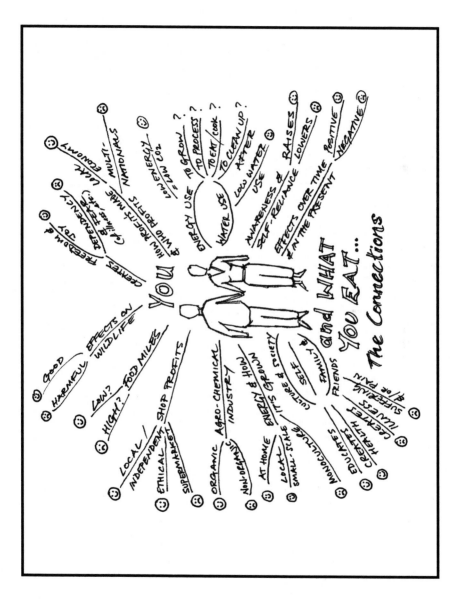

In the context of the development of humanity and civilisation, we are where we are – obviously. So I feel that as a first step we need to understand how to live in a changing and challenging world. I feel we need to become much more confident about dealing with this. And this is where both permaculture and confidence about our health are so, so critical.

If we want to move on and create sustainability and a more fulfilling quality of life, the best way to do this is to understand the nature of the world and to live harmoniously and creatively with it – to understand that we are a part of the web of life, not separate from it.

What do you see when you take a look at the future we are heading towards? Does it feel safe and secure? Does it feel good? Would you like to feel safer and more secure about your future and the future of the world as a whole?

A philosophy that treats all life with compassion and respect is not a romantic 'back to nature' view of the world; it is massively practical and utterly logical. It is not based on the idea that we should go back to anything, or on some view that everything was 'ever-so-nice' many centuries ago when we were all closer to the monkeys!

A philosophy of working with nature is all about the practicalities of how we go forward now. It is about how we work with the creative, productive energy of life and nature to meet our own needs, by understanding the needs of our children, the next generation, and the next seven generations (to borrow a Native American way of thinking). Working with nature is a practical way of life that is rooted in the realisation that the way we think and act now does create our future. For me, its deepest roots are in a sense of nature and evolution that is beyond words. As a philosophy and way of life it seeks balance, harmony, diversity, abundance, beauty and natural, organic growth – a balance of intellect and intuition. In fact it doesn't even seek these... it just works with the natural flows, patterns and energies that naturally create these desirable outcomes. Working with nature means, for example, a recognition that creating beauty in what we do is really, really good for us in a practical sense, and is therefore very important.

Working with nature means working with all forms of nature, including our own. It does not mean using 'human nature' as an excuse for our destructive and not so desirable behaviour. It means recognising and building on the creative and inspirational nature of our behaviour. Nature is always changing, and constantly growing. We always have the capacity to learn and change.

For me, our nature inevitably includes an evolutionary element. For most of our 'civilised' history it has been accepted that civilising ourselves includes an evolution of our values. Legal and religious systems, and spiritual philosophies have been developed to uphold the values that were seen to be 'right' and proper at the time by certain people. Evolution doesn't stop, so I feel that our thinking and values should still be evolving – and naturally I see nature as our best guide for this type of conscious evolution.

Where do you see our values going in the present age of civilisation? Do you feel we are making progress in creating a more caring world?

Personally, I feel that respecting all forms of life, human, animal and plant life is important. To me 'Thou shalt not kill' means 'Thou shalt not kill' – which means no killing at all. And you really need to sit with this to sense what it really means – which has little to do with simplistic interpretations of the Bible!

I do not feel that these values makes me 'better' than some one that does kill, or some one that eats meat. However, I do feel 'better' in myself, although not in a smug way. I feel it is better for me, myself, and for my relationship with the web of life. I have also found that not eating meat or animal products is a surprisingly easy and enjoyable step along my path towards a more compassionate way of life.

Inevitably, such issues are personal choices which depend on the particular information, guidance and experiences we chance upon or seek out along our life's path. I know that I now feel better informed in my choices – my inner feelings and confidence about those choices are also much stronger.

A Route to Personal and Planetary Health?

The combination of a wider understanding of raw food and permaculture is a serious yet playful, semi-subversive yet utterly democratic route to creating individual and community health, greater freedom, and much greater self-reliance and self-confidence. But then again, what's subversive about love and compassion, life, nature and health creation?

I see sustainable living as being about enabling the head and heart to be integrated. The life, the environment and the relationships that we create around us all come through our thoughts and values. Once we see, feel or understand this, then we start to sense how a more sustainable lifestyle can be created. We really understand how the health of one depends on the health of the other – there is no separation. And without it we get nowhere, fast.

At the moment we often place the responsibility for sustainability and health outside ourselves; with the government, the doctors, the drug companies and the health service. Government policy and the medical establishment will never create health, because they maintain a dependency culture that is inevitably self-justifying and which completely accepts and believes in high levels of sickness as 'normal'. Unhealthy foods happen to be very costly for our health, whilst also being profitable for the drug and medical industry and the food processing industry. I don't think many people knowingly make others sick for profit – it just happens to be a cycle that our very clever yet equally unwise society is locked into because we don't seem to know any better. And that's because we don't have any well used routes for learning from nature, which is in turn because as a modern, developed, scientific society we tend to think we know better than nature. We observe nature, watching it on TV or reading about it endlessly, but we don't really 'know' it anymore, because our own nature has become so distorted. We are offered little real choice, because most of the choices we are offered are inevitably hooked into the great consumption-directed global marketing machine in some way or other.

I know that some people do think there is more to the current state of human and planetary health than just chance. If you take away someone's health you take away a large part of their freedom – think about it. In this way you can create a population that lives in fear of sickness, disease and death. So the fear leads to a dependency on working to earn money, to pay for the health insurance, the medical care, the distractions that are needed to hide the fear, and so on. Some might suggest that a population that is 'dumbed down' with heavy and addictive foods is easier to manipulate and exploit. So I've heard some people say in a jokey yet totally serious way to those that do believe in conspiracy theories "You aren't going to eat more of that conspiracy food are you?". If you are into conspiracy theories or even corporate and governmental collusion then take a look at food and health – or rather, illness. If that's the sort of thing you believe in then you might just find one of the biggest potential conspiracies going. Try starting a positive health creating conspiracy to balance things out, and start with yourself... it is the only place you can start in fact.

Whatever you think, the point is that if you want health you have to create it for yourself. And we can all achieve this once we understand the nature of health. For me this has been very empowering. So in creating individual and community health and freedom we can break the dependency culture that is justified and maintained by peoples understandable fears of illness and disease, which typically gets greater as people get older, or as they start to find they are sick. We can also transform an economy that profits from ill-health and the products that create disease. And by using permaculture we can become much more able and confident in meeting our own needs – which again helps to overcome the dependency culture and creates empowered and self-reliant individuals and communities.

Thriving by Meeting Our Needs

In developing our ideas about our needs, most theory and practice in psychology has built up by studying people who suffer disturbed behaviour or mental illness. Abraham Maslow took a perhaps radical step by concentrating on healthy and fully functioning individuals![15] He then assessed what people's needs seemed to be in this healthy state. Maslow's humanistic picture of healthy human needs therefore differs considerably from the behaviourists and virtually all of the rest of preceding psychological theory and practice. His description of healthy human needs is summarised as follows:

---

[15] It is worth pondering for a moment about how things might change if our medical research studied physical health and health creation much more than they studied illness and disease.

* Physiological Needs: Biological needs for oxygen, food, water and suitable body temperature. These are the strongest needs – without them we die.

* Safety Needs: Adults experience these needs in periods of disruption, children experience them much more continually.

* Love, Affection and Belongingness Needs: Needs to avoid loneliness and alienation, and needs to give and receive love, affection and belonging.

* Esteem Needs: Self-respect and respect from others, required for confidence in our thinking and action. Without these people feel inferior, weak, helpless and worthless.

* Self-Actualisation: For Maslow this is the individual achieving what she or he was born to do. It is fulfilling a 'calling'. Without movement towards this the person is restless and something is just not quite right with the world.

Our pursuit of growth based, scientific and technological development is leaving many of these needs unmet. Therefore it makes sense to look for sustainable ways to meet each of the needs within Maslow's hierarchy. What kind of individuals, families, communities and society would we have if we actually did prioritise these needs, and used the economy intelligently to meet these needs? What good reason is there not to aim for this, and not to start acting as if we want and deserve these things for ourselves and others now? So why not start now!?

Our body and mind emerged, producing our uniquely sophisticated brain and consciousness, from a raw, evolutionary soup (or more likely a fruit salad!) that met all our needs. It must have met all those needs because that 'soup' enabled our unique human consciousness to emerge. Generally what we eat now is very, very different from that evolutionary soup. Scientifically we know that this change must have an effect – both in each of our life times and from one generation to the next generation. So that creates subtly different humans, that don't fit the original, evolutionary blueprint.

To what extent does our current diet meet our needs for the optimum functioning of our complete mind-body-consciousness? How can we have any realistic idea of our genuine needs unless we actually experience different diets and lifestyles?

The only genuine knowledge of how our needs are being met comes from what we experience. Anything else is just ideas in our head, that create an illusion of knowing which is actually based on 'ideas about' something rather than real experience. And the point is that unless you try eating more raw foods then you will never actually know its effects – although you will have plenty of ideas about its effects. Unless you try it over a long enough period of time, in a well informed way, you will never know the effects over time. And you will never find out if your ideas are right or misinformed.

I have found a raw food diet immensely liberating in many ways. It is still unusual in our society, so it generates interest, and some people do see it as odd or weird (which I find weird because it just feels so natural to me!). However, because my choices are based on good information, personal experience and a strong, good feeling, I feel free of what people might think about me. This is common amongst raw food eaters.

I can see that if enough of us go for more raw food and permaculture, people will start to notice, and as a result the economy and society will then change. People notice how healthy and alive raw foodies are. As a lifestyle it is already becoming more widely known and understood, and therefore seen as more normal. We don't have to talk about it – although many do because of the joy, energy and enthusiasm it has brought them, and because it feels so strange that so few people know about it. The same goes for permaculture.

Sustainable Living

I feel that combining bodily intuition with the practical whys and hows of permaculture offers us opportunities to create many benefits for people and planet in meeting our hierarchy of needs. This means both enjoying a balanced health creating diet and designing a productive and beautiful landscape in which to live.

Once again, think about the effects on the global ecosystem, and local ecosystems, if we stopped eating so much wheat[16] and other foods that create lifeless and degrading environments, and ate fruit and tree crops, which would be good for you too.

The thoughts and values that are embodied in a philosophy of working with nature can free blockages that create stress or prevent action. This improves health and allows thinking to flow naturally with action because there is an inner knowing that is in accord with principles of healthy, sustainable living. When 'being' in this way all the words, theory and ideas are a long way away. Things just flow; the inner feeling of trust and knowing is there and it guides the way without the mind jabbering away, trying to control everything and getting in the way of direct experience.

A key to open the door to individual health and sustainability is to understand how you understand – and then to use that understanding to create systems around you that generate health and sustainability. You can then design systems through which nature's beautiful, harmonious, health creating processes can flow. This may mean creating some mental image or feeling for how things can change. Or it may mean allowing your body

[16] See the book *Grain Damage* by Dr Douglas Graham, available through Healthful Living International – contact details are in the appendices section of this book.

to inform your mind which are foods that are health creating foods – really feeling the effects of different tastes in your mouth and foods in your body. It means taking responsibility for our own patterns of thinking and values, as well as our systems of growing or buying food, systems of gaining a living, and systems of involvement with other people, so that these are all in harmony with nature.

This might sound very rational stuff to some – or it might sound like some kind of romanticised fantasy to others. I hope it will feel good, and strike a chord with many. And I hope it reflects the vision of others.

A harmonious and compassionate way of life is at its strongest and is often very powerful when you let go of the rational and go with the flow; at its most beautiful when there is no busy, busy thinking; action in harmony with nature. Conflict and friction rapidly start to dissolve because there is no need to understand or control – inner trust and inner knowing create inner peace and harmonious action.

An amazing amount can be achieved when thinking and actions are in accord with nature. And this includes the amazing things that happen when we get out of the way and allow nature's innate intelligence (which is part of all of us) to create better levels of health for us. The ultimate goal is to have no friction between self and universe; living in accord with creation, not fighting it or trying to control it.

✳ Can you see yourself living in healthy and natural harmony?

✳ What might it feel like?

If you do not feel drawn to a high percentage raw diet, and do not wish to give up meat or dairy produce, or wheat, at least think about the impacts and benefits of reducing meat, dairy and wheat consumption, and eating more raw foods or shifting to about 50% raw. Think about the impacts out there, in the wider world, as well as in your own life. At least feel free and confident about having a go from time to time. Flexibility and adaptability in diet and lifestyle all help to reduce our dependency, and increase our self-reliance.

Three keys to healthy and sustainable living:

UNDERSTANDING THE NATURE OF UNDERSTANDING

UNDERSTANDING THE NATURE OF HEALTH

UNDERSTANDING THE NATURE OF NATURE

Working With Nature In Diet:
Observation and Evolution As Our Guides

My choices about what I eat have changed significantly – in fact several of my 'reality tunnels' have been blown apart since I started to eat a high percentage of raw food in my diet. I choose to eat as I do now having eaten an omnivorous diet (with lots of meat) for the first 26 years of my life. I have also been both vegetarian and a non-evangelical vegan, for 3 years each (i.e. I just got on and did it).

For me a high percentage raw food diet includes Robert Hart's[17] 'R70 forest garden diet' (70% raw fruit, 'sallets'[18] and nuts/seeds), the hygienist approach promoted by Fred Paténaude, Dave Klein, Dr Douglas Graham, Professor Rozalind Gruben and many others, as well as 100% fruitarian, the 'living foods' diet as described by Elaine Bruce and Sibila's nature-guided, very simple and more intuitive approach (see later sections[19]).

Generally in raw food nutrition and in permaculture there are no rigid laws, although there are flexible guidelines, which you should be aware of. In raw food nutrition this includes sensible food combining, eating a low protein diet, and having a reasonable balance of fruits and vegetables, with limited eating of nuts and seeds. In the long term some of these diets seem to be more natural than others. Many people try the fruitarian option at some time, but few sustain it. The same goes for the living foods diet. In my experience these are good things to try, and they can have benefits, although in the longer term the balanced fruit and veg approach, with simple (simply delicious!) meals is the most likely one you'll settle into.

Intuitively I feel that a diet that consists of mainly raw fruit and veg, nuts and seeds is a 'more natural diet' for us. And logically, based on a great deal of evidence I have seen, heard and read, I also think that it is our most natural diet. Much of this book aims to show why I *think and feel* this is the case... as you are discovering I hope.

To explore what is a natural diet we need some guidelines on how nature works. Permaculture can provide these guidelines because it aims to mimic nature by ensuring that as far as is possible the needs of one part of the system (e.g. food growing), in some way will be meeting the needs of other elements in the system (e.g. you). This is relevant to diet because what you eat builds, maintains and fuels your own bodily living system (body-mind -spirit); and it is also relevant (because permaculture is about designing and creating ecologically

---

[17] Robert Hart is a wonderful gentleman whose ideas on forest gardening have had a major impact on the British permaculture movement – in particular through his books *Forest Gardening* and *Beyond the Forest Garden*.

[18] As described in *John Evelyn's Acetaria*: a discourse on sallets, originally published in 1699.

[19] You may also come across the 'instincto' philosophy. The vegan instincto's I have come across seem quite balanced people – those that follow the raw meat eating instincto philosophy on the other hand are following a clever bunch of severely distorted ideas, which has definitely shown in the distorted behaviour and physical and mental health of any of these 'carnivorous' instinctos that I have met.

sustainable, efficient and productive systems, and about designing ecological lifestyles[20]. So if we are to be consistent in using permaculture it is relevant to look at our own 'natural' mind-body-spirit system; our internal ecology).

A permaculture based high percentage raw diet represents working with nature because it is rooted in an understanding of life's processes and our basic natural needs. All life, including human life, the life in a soil, woodland or forest, is a regenerative, health building process – that is its nature, and nature naturally creates health.

Our body is a flow, it regenerates itself naturally. What we eat is a key factor in shaping how and with what we regenerate ourselves. We all know "you are what you eat". Most of our body is water, and over 95% of our cells are replaced within one year[21]. In seven years virtually every cell in our body has changed – we are literally a different person.

If we want to be healthy it makes sense to regenerate and replace those cells with the best possible materials, fuels and lubricants. Unlike many cooked foods, raw foods encourage, rather than hinder, the body's natural healing and regenerative process – they work with nature not against it.

Raw foods are rich in vital water, whilst many cooked foods are dehydrated or dehydrating. The natural way our digestive system works means that 'the juice is the food'– a phrase used by David Wolfe and others that is worth remembering. This means that ultimately all nutrition, yes *all* nutrition, comes into our body in liquid form through the walls of the digestive system. Therefore liquid rich whole raw organic plant foods such as fruits, leaves and vegetables form the very best vehicles for transporting these essential life giving, health creating minerals, vitamins and enzymes into our body. They require less work for the body to take in that nutrition. And they represent a flow of life giving energy.

Drinking good quality water is also beneficial to creating health and vitality as it helps flush unwanted toxins out of our cells. So remember, even as an adult, your body is a flow, rather than an unchanging object.

* If you want to understand how diet and lifestyle can create health you need to generate a vision of how your body works as a flowing system, a cleansing, healing river of life, a health creating process.

* You need to feel that it is your body's nature to create health, and sense how you can work with nature to create that health.

In understanding how to create health there are some very basic facts about the nature of our body's needs, and the nutritional nature of raw foods that are very useful to know. Firstly, Dr Douglas Graham – a long term raw fooder, ex-Olympic trampolenist, and professional training and health adviser to top

---

[20] This is the British permaculture teacher Stephen Nutt's simple and useful definition of permaculture.

[21] Dr Deepak Chopra, *Ageless Body, Timeless Mind*, Random House Audiobooks.

athletes – highlights some key facts that nutritionists accept; these facts are that of the conventionally accepted food groups:

* Fresh raw FRUITS are the very best source of VITAMINS and the second best source of minerals.

* Fresh raw VEGETABLES are the very best source of MINERALS and the second best source of vitamins.

Therefore, eating plenty of fresh raw fruit and fresh raw vegetables ensures that your diet will be well supplied from the best two sources of vitamins and minerals. It's that simple. And you don't need to buy a bunch of expensive pills and potions to get the best – you just have to understand that nature knows best, and buy or grow her vitamin and mineral packages... they're called fruits, vegetables, nuts and seeds.

In addition, fruit contains plenty of purified water as well as all its nutrients, so it is a great body cleanser. Meanwhile the chlorophyll that is in green leafy vegetables is a wonderful healer and rebuilder of the body. And it is a fascinating fact that chlorophyll is virtually identical in chemical structure to the haemoglobin in our blood – they are identical except that our haemoglobin is built around an iron molecule, whilst chlorophyll is centred on a magnesium molecule.

A second set of facts is emphasised in particular by David Wolfe and his colleagues in the dynamic organisation Nature's First Law. This is the nutritional triangle, or 'Sunfood Triangle':

It may seem a surprise but green leafy vegetables are the best foods for obtaining the proteins we need to build and maintain our body. This is because they contain the essential amino acids, minerals and vitamins that enable the body to build the proteins it needs – this is explained in more detail in the section 'the Protein Question' later. Green leaves are also the most alkaline of foods, which is extremely important and beneficial – and which is also explained later in the Acid - Alkaline Balance section.

David Wolfe's book *The Sunfood Diet Success System* is one of the best sources for understanding the key role of mineral rich foods, and therefore the importance of green leafy vegetables in a health creating diet. David Wolfe is also one of the leading raw food advocates with a deep understanding of the environmental benefits of eating a high raw plant food diet. For example he points out that raw plant foods are by far the most naturally abundant foods on the planet, therefore by eating much more of these naturally abundant foods we place much, much lower demands on nature and the environment.

Fruits and vegetables are the very best sources for the vitamins, minerals and sugars we need; and seeds, nuts and avocados are the best sources for the fats we need, with organic cold pressed oils being a useful back up. Sprouted pulses and seeds, such as alfalfa, chickpeas, green lentils, mung and so on are also packed with vital proteins, enzymes, vitamins and minerals. So by making sure we have an appropriate balance of these three essential food types, the ideal source of which is raw foods, we meet all our body's essential needs with ease. If your body as a flow is made up of health creating foods, it will naturally create health; you won't have to work for it.[22] But what is the right balance? Well – the answers to that question will be revealed as you read on!

By considering diet from a permaculture perspective, we can sense how matter and energy flow through us. Matter in some forms creates health in your body, and matter in other forms creates sickness. Looking at foods as flows of matter and energy, we can more easily see the many relationships that that matter and energy has with the outer world. Then we can gain an idea of how those relationships can be used to create and support personal and ecological health.

With this in mind the following section starts, firstly, by asking what permaculture is, and secondly, by asking: how is permaculture design and its underlying philosophy relevant to diet?

What is Permaculture?

Permaculture is not a static, fixed thing; it is an evolving set of ideas and lifestyles, and a movement concerned with the impacts and pleasures that are created from the way we live. It has been described as applied common sense, and the most useful of 'green' ideas. Basically it is a practical system of working out positive solutions to a whole range of questions. It is a practical philosophy and a set of tools and techniques for creating sustainable lifestyles that now, through this book and the development of permaculture that it offers, is being used to also create naturally healthy sustainable lifestyles too.

The term 'permaculture' comes from combining the ideas of permanent agriculture (including horticulture and silviculture) and permanent culture. Diet, food and nutrition is an important part of any culture – and inevitably it has to be a core concern for any permanent, sustainable culture.

"Permaculture is the conscious design and maintenance of agriculturally productive ecosystems which have the diversity, stability and resilience of natural ecosystems. It is the harmonious integration of landscape and people providing their food, energy, shelter, and other material and non-material needs in a sustainable way...

The philosophy behind permaculture is one of working with, rather than against, nature, of looking at systems in all their functions, rather than asking only one yield of them, and of allowing systems to demonstrate their own evolutions."

Bill Mollison, *Permaculture: A Designers' Manual*, Tagari Press, 1988.

Although many people who use permaculture advocate using domesticated animals within a permaculture system, permaculture ethics and principles

---

[22] These key processes are described in more detail in many books such as David Wolfe's *The Sunfood Diet Success System*, and Susie Miller's *Raw Food Nutrition*.

themselves do not. Permaculture ethics and principles are applied by different people in different ways. Permaculture is not owned by anyone – it was designed to be so by Bill Mollison, the initial creator of permaculture, with David Holmgren – this is one of its strengths. So I use permaculture as I wish to help create cruelty free, domesticated animal free systems... that are packed with wildlife. And I recommend that any vegans that think permaculture means using animals look again at the fundamental ethics and principles of permaculture – interpret them from your own perspective not someone else's! Don't get stuck with the idea that permaculture is the way that some people use it.

Permaculture can be an art or a science, a mental technology or a spiritually based philosophy – it is what you make it. It is a way of thinking and living that is about creating efficient, productive and sustainable systems, and about 'designing sustainable lifestyles'[23].

There are three fundamental permaculture ethics:

EARTH CARE

PEOPLE CARE

FAIR SHARE

These three ethics provide a good starting point for considering how we meet the needs of our own natural mind-body-spirit system. After considering these core ethics, we will look at the basic principles used in permaculture, and how they are relevant to diet.

Earth Care: Ecological Sustainability

In most climates where humans live, if left to do its own thing, nature will create a forest. So, in ecology, a woodland or forest is normally what's called the 'climax ecosystem'. These are generally the most productive land-based ecosystems in terms of biodiversity (variety and quantity of species) and plant biomass. Woodlands and forests are also very stable, and generally they create, maintain and protect the soil. They involve a whole lot of mutually beneficial and productive relationships between trees and other plants, animals, insects, bacteria, fungi, worms, soil and so on.

For me, Earth Care means care for all the Earth's living creatures because all creatures are part of the Earth's web of life. So I choose to avoid meat, dairy and other animal products. For me, it is preferable to create food producing habitats that supply the needs of both humans and wildlife. Knowing now that I do not need animal products to be fully healthy, forest gardening and agro-forestry seem to me to maximise care for the earth and all its inhabitants, as they are based on creating highly diverse, productive

---

[23] This is the simplest and most useful short definition of permaculture I know.

and stable forest and woodland ecosystems. They are ideal for a high percentage fruit or raw food diet, and for supplying many other needs such as timber and fibres, and are described in more detail later in this book.

I also believe that growing huge quantities of wheat and cereals needs looking at seriously when considering Earth Care. Whether grown for bread or for animal feeds, crops such as wheat and maize invariably create mono-cultural deserts as well as involving massive energy and agro-chemical use. Wheat was originally a plant that grew in the semi-desert areas of what was Persia; and to grow it we mimic its natural environment, i.e. we have created and now maintain and expand man-made deserts all around the world in order to grow wheat. So even organic bread depends on creating semi-deserts – and to me this is not an ideal strategy for Earth Care or sustainability!

The Romans massively extended the Sahara in north Africa because it was their wheat growing belt, and now we are doing the same all around the world. In contrast to wheat, fruit grows on trees, and salads can be grown as part of a forest garden. This involves a lot less work and other energy inputs and creates a diverse and stable habitat. That's what I call Earth Care! So long as you're not eating foods that have been transported half-way around the planet, a mainly or all raw diet is great for Earth Care – and all the more so when you're growing it yourself or buying locally.

Overall this ethic encourages working with nature and evolution to increase the overall productivity and diversity of nature, and thereby caring for the Earth by increasing its overall pool of life.

People Care: Meeting Human Needs

People Care is about meeting our own many and diverse needs – as individuals and groups – because if we are to care for the Earth we need to care for ourselves, as part of the Earth, rather than battling with the Earth to meet our needs.

By understanding that permaculture is about community, communication and lifestyle, as well as growing food and dealing with our wastes, we can see how it can be used to meet our many needs – physical needs, security needs, love, affection and belongingness needs, esteem needs and our needs for deeper fulfilment in life[24]. When left to do their thing, evolution and nature generally create healthy and fully functioning natural systems – health is nature's norm. Indeed, understanding this is the essence that permaculture is founded on. So to me it seems that if we want to maximise People Care, we want to create and maximise vibrant health in people – physical, mental, emotional and spiritual.

Physiologically a raw food diet tends to create a more alkaline body, which reduces bodily acidity and stress. In contrast, a more normal but less natural

[24] This is based on Abraham Maslow's *Hierarchy of Needs*.

high protein, high fat and artificial sugar diet creates an acid body, which increases physical and emotional tension and stress; which is hard for the person involved and for those around them. If you look around you in your life you will see that an acid body very often creates an acid personality!

Many of our society's major illnesses are strongly linked to diet. Our ability to fight illness and disease (our immune response) is directly linked to what we eat. Health is also a major factor that affects how people feel about their quality of life. Raw foods cleanse the body's systems. They strengthen the immune system and thereby support health and healing. They improve the quality of life for people, because they give people confidence about their health, with increased levels of vitality and mental clarity. As well as reducing the likelihood of illness and suffering for the person eating the healthier, more natural diet, it also reduces the likelihood of friends and family experiencing very real and significant emotional suffering as a result of a loved-one's illness. Acting to reduce the 'web of suffering' created by such high levels of illness and disease throughout our society is something I see as excellent People Care. Even if I alone take responsibility for my own health, then I am acting to avoid the suffering that loved ones might experience if I did become ill. Which is caring for those that care for me.

A high raw food diet also often leads to greater self-awareness, and can often generate a strong desire for networking, socialising and community because of wanting to be amongst others with a similar lifestyle and philosophy. Being in a community increases the number of beneficial relationships an individual can draw on to meet her or his needs. So in many, many ways a raw food, and permaculture lifestyle is a very powerful form of People Care.

Fair Share: Equity in Choice and Consumption, and Sharing of Surplus.

This is about fairness in resource consumption; it also means sharing surpluses. For me, Fair Share means everyone and everything having its basic needs met. Fair Share is also about:

* Being willing to work with nature to obtain our fair share of food, shelter and other needs, and to create a healthy and fulfilling lifestyle.

* Aiming to make sure that our lifestyle only uses our fair share of planetary resources – which means much less resources than a typical western diet and lifestyle require.

* Not playing a part in the exploitation of others – human or animal, plants, soils, landscape and habitats as a whole.

* Sharing our surpluses.

As the dynamic and environmentally aware American raw food advocate David Wolfe points out, raw plant foods are by far the most naturally abundant foods on the planet. So there are plenty of these foods for all, and nature clearly likes to provide foods as raw plant foods, because they are so abundant.

I believe that all life should have its fair share of resources. I know that a vegan, high percentage raw food permaculture diet, catered for by forest gardening, forest farming and permaculture can meet all my physical needs. So to me this diet feels like a fair and equitable way of meeting my human needs through ecologically positive food growing systems, that also leave a lot more land to be re-colonised by nature. Forest gardening and agroforestry[25] are ecologically efficient, effective, healthy and easily accessible ways to feed ourselves, whilst also catering for the needs of so many other living things.

To summarise my own experience of permaculture, I would say that in theory, and also in practice, it is about:

✳ Being really observant, in order to understand (sense, or get a feel for) and experience the nature of nature, the nature of evolution, the nature of consciousness, and how these inter-react and inter-relate; to understand our web of effects in the world.

✳ Based on this understanding/experience, it is about living a life that develops constructive, positive, healthy and beneficial relationships between elements of our living environment, our lifestyles and ourselves – including in the various elements of our selves (the inter-related mind-body-spirit, emotion system).

Summarising my own view on ethics and lifestyle, I know that many people do have strong ethics that significantly influence the lifestyle they choose to lead. If you have a sense of the sacredness of nature, planet earth, Gaia, Goddess, God, you will find that if you eat a higher proportion of raw plant foods you are building your bodily 'temple' from food that still contains a vibrant life force. Which contains more of the living energy of nature, planet earth, Gaia, Goddess, God, a crisp apple or fresh green salad, or a baked potato, bowl of steamed rice, a Big Mac or slice of roast meat? Certainly, any kind of highly processed food contains no life force at all. And if it contains no life force, then ask yourself 'what kind of force does it contain instead?'

What I suggest is that if you are an environmentalist, a 'green' or someone who deeply respects Gaia, and if you are a vegetarian or a vegan then you will find that eating at least 50% raw plant foods is completely in line with your ethics and values; it probably takes your ethics further in fact. It can only help you achieve more of what you want to achieve through the lifestyle choices you are already making.

---

[25] Agroforestry uses lots of tree crops and the benefits provided by trees (e.g. shelter from winds, mulch/green manure materials, nitrogen fixing, etc). Agroforestry and forest farming can use techniques such as alley cropping, where bushes, arable or market garden crops, etc are grown along alleys between fruit trees.

'Mollisonian' Permaculture Design Principles and their Relevance to Diet

Bill Mollison, the founder of Permaculture with David Holmgren, coined the following six principles as basic guides to permaculture thinking – they have become known to many as 'Mollisonisms'. In essence, these principles are ecological truisms that therefore can be used to guide, design and live a sustainable lifestyle. In the following paragraphs the Mollisonisms are applied to the consideration of growing and eating a high percentage raw food diet.

Work With Nature Not Against It

The principle of working with nature is simply based on the recognition that nature knows best when it comes to creating healthy, diverse and productive sustainable living systems.

There are many theories of human evolution, which when you step back and take a good look at them are all inevitably based on very limited evidence and a lot of guess work. Anatomically and physiologically we are scientifically categorised as 'great apes' and great apes are higher primates that evolved in the tropical forests. All other 'great apes' still live in tropical forests. Our natural characteristics suggest that for early humans forest dwelling came before our savannah stage. This is consistent with analysis of the wear and tear on early humans' teeth, and is also consistent with known facts about climate change that would have caused a shrinkage of the early 'humans' tropical forest home. My sense is that we mainly evolved in the forests and then we adapted to the savannah; so I feel that forest dwelling is our natural evolutionary home.[26]

As Dennis Nelson's excellent and very affordable little book *Maximizing Your Nutrition*[27] points out, zoologists have established five basic types of animals. These are based on their anatomy and physiology, and the obvious evolutionary adaptations, which clearly show how an animal's body is designed to specialise in eating particular foods in a certain environment:

Carnivores: feeding primarily on flesh, bones and blood; with claws, teeth or beaks for tearing, etc. e.g. big cats, buzzards, crocodiles, hyenas.

Herbivores: feeding primarily on grass or other vegetation. e.g. deer, cattle, elephants, bison, rabbits, horses.

---

[26] Not surprisingly archeologists will not have found any skeletons of our forest dwelling ancestors. Once you ask why, there are some pretty obvious answers. A tropical forest ecosystem, with all its mass of scavenging life, including ants, beetles and worms, would have broken down and disposed of any bodies and skeletons quickly and efficiently. And because archeologists are not ecologists they don't think about such obvious factors. So they have been convinced that we developed on the savannahs, basically because that's the only skeleton evidence they've found – which is understandable, but not really all that smart.

[27] Dennis Nelson, *Maximizing Your Nutrition*, 1988 – available from D. Nelson, Box 2302, Santa Cruz, California. 95063, USA.

Graminivores: feeding primarily on grains and seeds, e.g. many birds and rodents.

Omnivores: feeding on a mixed diet of plants, roots and flesh, e.g. pigs, bears, badgers, the dog family, etc.

Frugivores: feeding primarily on fruit and vegetation e.g. all primates such as lemurs, various monkeys, baboons, and the four species of 'anthropoid apes' – gorillas, chimpanzees (including bonobos), orangutangs and gibbons. Plus the fruit eating parrots – which evolved, eating only fruit, to be the most intelligent and long lived of all bird species.

Our physiology determines our natural capacity to get nutrients out of our food. And in his attempts to help people to understand that all animals on the earth are perfectly designed to eat a specific diet – including humans – American raw food educator Loren Lockman points out that technically speaking the term 'fruitarian' has no real meaning. On the other hand the term frugivore does have scientific meaning in relation to the natural diet for a body.

The fundamental point is that every creature on the planet gets everything it needs to be completely healthy if it eats its natural diet. So all we have to do is work out what our natural diet is if we want to know what foods will create and maintain natural health.

If you take a look at the size and shape of your guts, your teeth, your fingers, your eyes, your digestive juices and saliva, and so on, in a scientific, zoological way what do you find? You find that your 'canine teeth' or incisors are far smaller than those of chimpanzees and other primates – which suggests what? It indicates that even within the anthropoid apes we are the least adapted for meat eating. The design of your canine teeth is in effect useless as far as meat eating is concerned, and you also don't have the really big hard-wearing grinding molars needed for a diet of tough leaves and grains.

As a human, you have long intestines and low-acidity digestive juices that are not at all suited to meat eating. You do not have claws; you have delicate fingers suited to delicate picking and peeling. What's more you have a massive brain and very sophisticated digestive system that can get enough energy out of a couple of ripe bananas for you to be able to cycle for a couple of hours.

Looking beyond the body you certainly will not find any fossilised cookers or microwaves in our ancient human habitats! So, like our primate relatives, but even more so than most of them, zoologically all the evidence points directly towards your human body having evolved to be suited by nature to eat a raw mainly fruit diet, with some leaves. So physiologically we are primarily frugivores. Which means we can get everything that we need for complete health from our natural diet... which is mainly fruit.

On the other hand, we have to process grains to be able to eat them. Therefore they are not a natural food for us.

Most of us know that the healthiest and healing foods are fruit and various other raw foods – that's what we bring in to hospitals for sick friends and

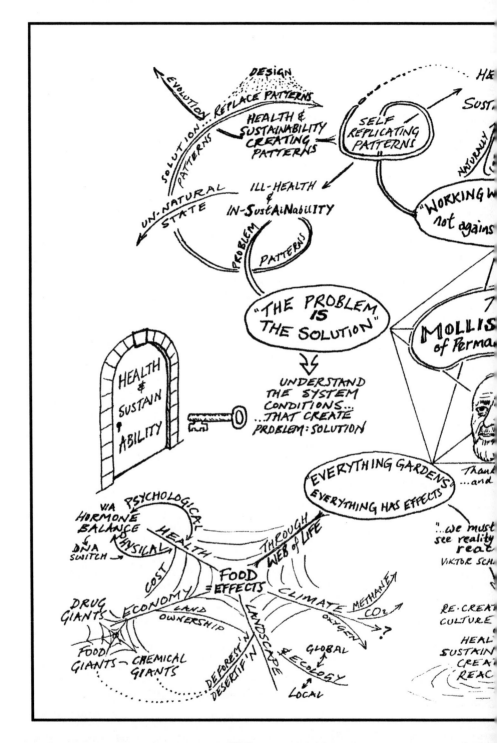

EVOLUTION

DESIGN
SOLUTION... REPLACE PATTERNS

HEALTH &
SUSTAINABILITY
CREATING
PATTERNS

SELF
REPLICATING
PATTERNS

HE

SUST

NATURALLY

UN-NATURAL STATE

PATTERNS

ILL-HEALTH
& IN-SustAiNabilITY

"WORKING W
not agains

PROBLEM
PATTERNS

"THE PROBLEM
IS
THE SOLUTION"

MOLLIS
of Perma

HEALTH
&
SUSTAIN
ABILITY

UNDERSTAND
THE SYSTEM
CONDITIONS...
...THAT CREATE
PROBLEM:SOLUTION

Thank
...and

"EVERYTHING GARDENS"
EVERYTHING HAS EFFECTS

VIA PSYCHOLOGICAL
HORMONE
BALANCE
&
DNA
SWITCH →

HEALTH

PHYSICAL

THROUGH
WEB OF LIFE

"..we must
see reality
rea
VIKTOR SCH

COST

FOOD
= EFFECTS

CLIMATE METHANE
CO2

RE·CREAT
CULTURE

DRUG
GIANTS

ECONOMY

LAND
OWNERSHIP

OXYGEN

?

HEAL
SUSTAIN
CREA
REAC

FOOD
GIANTS

CHEMICAL
GIANTS

LANDSCAPE

DEFOREST'N
DESERTIF'N

ECOLOGY

GLOBAL

LOCAL

NATURAL STATE →

NATURAL SYSTEMS — EVOLVE TOWARDS →

MULTI-LAYERED DIVERSE FOREST or WOODLAND (((HEALTHY)))

THAT CREATES →

PEOPLE HEALTH IN & FOR PLANET

CREATE DESIGN — MULTI-LAYERED DIVERSE LIFE

NATURALLY

CHANGE WHAT YOU EAT

CHEM. IND. AGRICULTURE DRUG IND. SUPER-MKTS ECOLOGY HEALTH ETC.

HUGE RIPPLE EFFECT

"LEAST CHANGE FOR MOST EFFECT" Max Output for Min. Effort

UNHEALTHY & UNSUSTAINABLE →

HEALTHY & SUSTAINABLE

CREATING MONOCULTURES: SAVANNAH & SEMI-DESERT

CREATING MORE AGRO-FORESTRY & FOREST GARDENS

SICKNESS CREATING FOOD & ECONOMY OF AGRO-CHEM, FOOD & DRUG GIANTS

HEALTH CREATING FOOD & ECONOMY OF ORGANICS & LOCAL FOOD LINKS

YIELD IS UNLIMITED (theoretically) by nature & evolution

DEPENDS ON

CLIMATE COMPANIONS

NATURE & NICHE EVOLUTION

UNDERSTANDING OF

FOOD SHELTER MATERIALS ENERGY BEAUTY 'GROWTH'

MIND — SPIRIT — "NEEDS" — EMOTION — BODY

PLANT NEEDS

HARMONIOUS BALANCE OF NEEDS & OUTPUTS

PLANT NEEDS

relatives. But to live on that really healthy raw fruit and veg alone...?

In peeling off hundreds of years of social, psychological and physiological conditioning as well as my own preconceptions, my research and experience of the issues suggests that eating and growing for a high percentage fruit and raw food diet definitely works with nature more than any other way of life.

In the UK and temperate climates, we are clearly not able to grow a tropical fruit diet for ourselves. However, with knowledge of permaculture and a true science of nutrition, we can grow a wide variety of fruits, leaves and vegetables that bring us closer to our natural evolutionary diet, whilst also creating personal and ecological health.

Fruit was designed by nature specifically to be attractive to eat, because it is the way that fruiting plants spread seeds and ensure their survival and evolution. No other 'food' is designed by nature to be eaten in such a wholly positive way; in fact many normal foods have to be cooked to remove the toxins that nature has put in them to stop them being eaten. Fruit is packed full of things that are good for its eaters; nature rewards fruit eaters with delicious sweetness and wonderful flavours. So the fruit eaters have a lovely and enjoyable time eating the fruit, they spread the seed, and with the smaller seeds they do the fertilising job all at the same time! So eating fruit, that nature designed to be eaten without harming or harvesting a whole tree, plant or animal, is definitely about working with nature.

Everything Gardens: - everything naturally creates the environment it needs, and everything has effects on and in the system:

Everything that is part of a system affects the nature and balance of that system – some things positively, some things negatively. Permaculture suggests that it makes good sense to work with the relationships that create positive effects, and to understand and avoid those that create negative effects. So in this sense, if you see your body as a garden, every food you 'plant' in it will influence the system as a whole, in a positive or negative way – both inside and out.

So wheat needs an acid environment in the body to be digested, so it creates an acid system. And for wheat to grow it needs deserts, which we busily create around the world for it, and have done since Greek and Roman times, doing far more work for wheat than it does for us in return – a realisation that has stuck with me since my first introduction to permaculture course.

All foods have some kind of influence on us; so they all 'garden' within our mind-body-spirit and emotional system. For example, to understand about the difference between raw and cooked food, it will be helpful to understand and remember the following important fact, which is well known amongst 'raw foodies' (this is one of the key scientific facts in this book and many other raw food books). Research in the 1930s discovered that raw foods and cooked foods have one particular difference in the way the body responds to them. Scientists at the Institute of Clinical Chemistry in Lausanne discovered a natural response called 'digestive leucocytosis'[28] which involves the body responding to all cooked foods as foreign (i.e. unnatural) matter. This reaction involves a major response from the immune system when cooked foods enter the body, which sends a rush of white blood cells – leucocytes – to the intestines to deal with this foreign matter coming in. This occupies the immune system and makes it less able to fight other bodily invaders. This immune response does not happen with raw foods. Think about that for a moment.

This raises one of the critical points about raw foods. And that is that cooking changes the chemical composition of foods. Raw foods are built of chemicals that have been created by nature, and therefore the body has an ability to recognise them. Cooked foods, and particularly highly processed foods[29], contain a much, much greater variety of chemical compounds because the heating and processing change the nature of the natural chemicals and creates many more chemical compounds. The body has no natural ability to recognise these chemicals – which is why it recognises them as foreign matter and has the immune response mentioned above. Some of these chemical concoctions it will do its best to throw out straight away, but many others get stored in the body – particularly in the fats – and gradually have a degenerating effect because they don't have a natural role in the body; so they clog it up, influence the growth of cells in an unnatural way or have some other unnatural effect.

Natural, health creating foods create a body that will give them what they want and need, which is a healthy vibrant body that can efficiently and effectively digest and assimilate them and spread their seed.

Raw food permaculture works with the foods that have positive health creating effects, and it avoids foods that have negative effects. This philosophy is pure permaculture. In contrast, most cooked foods act rather like agrochemicals – they do a job but their damaging effects are well hidden. You can't actually see the agrochemicals in non-organic food and you can't actually see the toxins in fried and processed foods – they are well hidden, but they do have a long term effect.

It's also worth considering 'economic gardening', or where and how you spend your money. Each time you spend your money it's like watering or feeding a plant. It feeds some kind of economic entity, which then spreads down through a web to its suppliers, employees, managers, owners and so on. If you buy local and organic you are feeding good 'plants' and a positive chain or web in the economy; if you are not, then you are feeding something less beneficial and potentially harmful to the overall welfare of the ecosystem. Buy consciously – and grow your own too, on your own or with others.

My observation and experience tell me that within a largely raw diet, and

---

[28] See digestive leucocytosis in Susannah and Leslie Kenton's *The New Raw Energy*, Vermillion, 1994, pages 41 & 89.

[29] This includes junk foods of course, which includes crisps, as well as convenience snacks, pre-cooked meals, microwave meals, most biscuits, cakes and sweets, canned and bottled drinks, and so on.

with intelligent use, different types of fruit and raw foods can be used to tackle illness and promote natural health, at both a personal and planetary level. Creating forest gardens and agroforestry systems to provide those foods involves creating stable and productive ecosystems that to a large extent garden themselves. Everything we eat has an effect, both inside us and outside us through its chain of effects. Toxic foods create and maintain a toxic environment for themselves in our bodies, healthy foods create healthy cells and a healthy environment in our bodies.

Minimum Effort for Maximum Effect

This principle is about understanding systems and seeing how the maximum beneficial effect can be achieved with minimal changes.

Fruit and other raw foods work with nature to produce maximum health with little effort. They also require less work to prepare and clean up after, tend to reduce or remove processing, cut right down on packaging and containers, require no use of energy or other resources in cooking and do not destroy the food value of vitamins, enzymes, etc. For proper digestion and assimilation of all the nutrients in foods we need vitamins, minerals *and* enzymes to work together – in effect they are what's called a 'guild'[30], which is normally where plants and trees benefit each other and work together in a group. So vitamins, minerals and enzymes are a 'nutritional guild', so that the whole effect of them working together is definitely greater than the sum of its constituent parts.

We need a range of essential amino acids in our diet to be strong and healthy[31]. Cooking kills the enzymes in food that are vital for assimilation of amino acids as most food enzymes are destroyed above about 42°C. Cooking food requires more work in processing and preparation, much more careful storing to keep it 'safe' to eat, far more work in clearing up, and you get much less out of your food because you've killed all those enzymes and depleted the vitamins and minerals – so cooked food usually = more effort + less effect! Which is not in line with basic permaculture principles at all.

And just in case anyone is wondering, there is a huge amount of pleasure that arises from eating more natural raw foods because the body loves to eat what it is naturally designed to eat. It sometimes takes a while to adjust as the taste and pleasure systems are cleaned up, but nature and evolution definitely designed pleasure into the equation.

Because it is designed to be eaten, if it is ripe[32] most fruit tastes delicious and

---

[30] 'Guilds' are defined and described in more detail in a later section.

[31] For a list of essential amino acids, and good food sources for them, see p.49 *Feel Good Foods* (Miller and Knowler), Susie Miller's *Raw Food Nutrition* booklet or any other good raw food book.

[32] And please note that ripeness is very important; it is the state fruit is naturally meant to be eaten in. Please also note that supermarkets are just about the worst place to go if you want to know what ripe fruit tastes and feels like. Unripe fruit leads to less losses, and easier handling; and people still buy it because they don't know any better, and have virtually no choice of ripe fruit in a supermarket. There's service for you!

only takes about half an hour to digest on an empty stomach. This means the body uses less energy in digesting fruit (and doesn't spend energy and resources on the immune response mentioned earlier). In contrast, cooked foods require a lot of work and energy to break down and digest, particularly when different food types are combined. Vegan raw food/fruitarian waste (bodily and through food preparation) also takes less work to create a safe compost, because it is less over-loaded with toxins and pathogens.

Via the food chain, all animal protein is built from the fruit/vegetable based amino acids that are the basic building blocks of life. However, on average, it takes about 10 kilos of vegetable protein to build 1 kilo of meat protein – this does not mean we are getting ten times as much from meat. It does mean that it takes at least ten times more land and water, fertilisers and energy, to create 1 kilo of meat protein. As part of an edible ecosystem it is much more efficient, in terms of land, energy and so on, to obtain amino acids direct from plants than it is to take them from animal protein.

So there are many, many ways that growing and eating more raw plant foods produce a maximum positive effect, with minimum effort.

Yield is Theoretically Unlimited

In theory, adjustments can always be made to a system to increase its yield.

There needs to be more exploration of the multiple benefits or yields that come to the mind-body-spirit, and to people and planet, from the adoption of lifestyles based on a high proportion of raw foods. The extent of the benefits will depend on information, skills and knowledge. The greatest long term benefits will arise as one generation passes a more complete health to the next, at conception and during pregnancy. I know raw children that are glowing examples of health, very bright, intelligent and happy; they suffer far less (and often not at all) from the supposedly 'normal' and seemingly unnecessary childhood colds and other illnesses that I suffered, and that I see most children suffering. I know of one raw eight or nine year old boy, raw from birth, who is one of the most balanced children I've met; enthusiastic but not 'hyper' or emotionally suppressed, and sensitive but not clingy and dependent (which obviously says a lot about his parenting too).

This does not mean that I believe a human breast milk and fruit/raw diet for babies automatically creates happy people – raising children is clearly far more complicated than that, with parental imprinting, natural nurturing, Continuum Concept factors[33], and other influences being highly important. (*The Mother* magazine is an excellent source of information and inspiration on these and other natural parenting issues – see Appendix 3.)

Optimum nutrition of mind, body, spirit and emotions is what we all need. Starting children off on that basis, in forest garden communities (including urban forest garden communities) with optimum nutrition (whatever you may

---

[33] See *The Continuum Concept*, Jean Liedloff – a very important book.

consider that to be), the benefits and 'yield' for them as individuals and for the communities they are part of would be enormous – both in the present and the future. This may not be easy to get started, but it can only become easier as more people explore what it means in practice.[34]

Harvest Only Sunshine

This principle is based on the realisation that ultimately all energy sources on the planet are derived from the sun's energy. Therefore it makes sense to shift to direct harvesting of that solar energy, via plants or appropriate technology. It is about 'closing the loop' – designing our lives, diets, and living systems so that all energy and resources are cycled back into nature, food production and organic growth.

A locally produced organic high percentage raw lifestyle seems to me to be the closest we can get to sustainable energy and resource use in our food production. Eating more raw foods clearly uses less or no energy for cooking. Some people do use processors and juicers. Personally I am naturally and happily moving to a more simple diet and I haven't used or needed a fridge for years, and obviously don't need a cooker or a freezer. My manual juicer, that will last a lifetime, is replacing the electric one, and the hand-mincer has replaced the blender, which is more enjoyable too.

The sun's energy combines with the energy of life to give us everything we need – vitamins, minerals, enzymes, amino-acids – in the best form, and the only ideal form. When will we learn nature's wisdom? We only really learn this aspect of natural, evolutionary wisdom when we experience it.

Fruit and chlorophyll are a direct harvest of sunshine. Fruit is sunlight turned directly into sugars and vitamins in particular, and green leaves are sunlight turned directly into chlorophyll and minerals in particular. So eating them fresh and raw is the most direct way for a human body to harvest only sunshine. What's more, positive responses to create health and sustainability improve vitality, self-reliance and quality of life – they create a harvest of smiley faces: human sunshine.

The Problem is the Solution

This for me, along with *working with nature*, is the most powerful of these attitudinal permaculture principles. If you get into permaculture they are positive attitudes that will become instilled in you. This principle is based on the realisation that the route to creating a real solution is to start by accepting and understanding the nature of the problem. It contains a deep wisdom, as well as great simplicity.

Levels of ill-health and disease, and the whole range of sustainability issues, are clearly significant 'problems' for our society. Einstein said that a society cannot solve a significant problem at the same level of thinking that created it; the society

[34] See the Appendices section for information about the Ecoforest community vision.

has to move to a new level of thinking. What does this mean in practice?

Diet, and the 'food' production, marketing and trading system, are clearly linked to a huge proportion of physical and psychological health problems, to exploitative economic systems, environmental destruction, and a considerable amount of animal suffering. So food and agriculture are central to health and sustainability problems – which also means that changing our thinking and our behaviour in these areas will lead us to the solutions. They will improve the quality of economic development and improve our quality of life.

It's actually quite simple:

* Many common foods that have to be cooked to be digestible help to create the problems – ill-health, soil depletion, desertification (i.e. wheat), erosion and pollution, releasing methane to the atmosphere to add to global warming (i.e. cattle and paddy fields).

* Many raw foods help create the solutions – health and sustainability, tree planting, stable soils, ground water retention and availability, trees binding carbon dioxide from the atmosphere.

We all have choices about the cause-and-effect food chain that we sit hungrily at the end of – which is also significantly influenced by the way we obtain our food. Which do you choose? Problem causing food chains, or solution causing food chains?

A poor diet is linked to a great deal of human suffering. There is the suffering of the sick themselves, often including physical, emotional or mental pain, as well as the stress, anguish and distress suffered by their family and friends. In wealthy nations this suffering often arises from avoidable lifestyle and diet related illness and disease, such as heart disease. In poorer nations this suffering is often caused by a lack of food, poor food in nutritional terms or a lack of dietary diversity. This is often worsened by wealthier nations and global institutions imposing inappropriate western agricultural practices upon the poorer nations, as conditions for gaining loans (i.e. debt) and so called 'aid'. It is also caused by western companies selling wholly inappropriate foods to the innocent – such as Nestlé's dreadful sales of artificial milk to nursing mothers in Africa.[35]

Kerala in southern India is an example of an alternative approach. Whilst Kerala is poor in income terms, it has very high literacy and has a highly productive forest garden system, as well as an economy that includes a large number of women's co-operatives.

Meanwhile, back in the west, it is now increasingly obvious that many of the wealthier nations are amongst the sickest nations in the world:

* Australians eat more red meat per head than any other nation – they also have the highest incidence of cancer.

* Americans consume more food per head and more dairy produce than any

---

[35] Contact the excellent Baby Milk Action campaign for more information – 23 St Andrew's Street, Cambridge CB2 3AX, UK.

other nation – they are the most obese (with about 50% of the population now overweight) and have the highest incidence of calcium deficiency.[36]

And there is not just human illness, there is the sickness imposed on ecosystems by our intensive, industrial agricultural practices too:

✳ Agro-industrial beef production uses 100,000 litres of water per 1kg of meat – that's about 10,000 gallons per lb!

✳ In Britain over 80% of arable land is used for growing animal fodder crops; and it takes about 10 kilos of vegetable or grain based animal protein to build 1 kilo of animal protein.

✳ To grow those animal fodder crops we put typically 10 times more energy into the food growing (fertiliser production and distribution, farm machinery fuels, harvesting and distribution, packaging, etc.) than we get out (in calories).

Based on facts like these, I see eating meat and dairy produce, and the traditional western diet[37] including high quantities of processed food products which rely on vast semi-desert and mono-cultures, as involving a great deal of unnecessary energy use, pollution and waste. At the same time they are actively reducing both human and ecological health – particularly in the long term (remember Pottenger's Cats?). The 'normal' diet and 'normal' agriculture seems like a very clear 'lose: lose' situation to me. In contrast, an organic high percentage raw diet generally promotes personal and planetary health – which is a 'win: win' situation.

Personally, on a Fair Share basis, I cannot justify being involved in taking the life of other creatures when I know I can easily meet my needs in other, more ecologically efficient ways. I believe that choosing to eat in a way that does not involve killing or cruelty is the positive path for ethical development and evolution.

The western agro-industrial and meat eating culture is used and abused by corporations that are spreading it around the world. This is creating short-lived grazing land where forests once were, and the dependence of people all over the world on single crops and genetically manipulated seeds, as well as costly pesticides and fertilisers supplied by multi-nationals. This destroys the self-reliance of developing countries, both agricultural and economic, and is consciously creating impoverishment, debt and dependency in order to sustain the global growth of trade, and the relative economic dominance of the developed nations.

There are other, much more loving ways to treat people and planet, that are also much more efficient and effective in meeting human needs e.g. forest garden and agroforestry systems.

The simplest and most direct way to stop your involvement in this destructive

---

[36] Source: Dr Joel Robbins, *Health Through Nutrition* audio tape.

[37] As many will know this is SAD in America – the Standard American Diet.

chain is a) to change what you eat, b) change how you get your food, and c) change who and where you get it from.

So, you need to grow at least some of your own food and/or buy it from local independent health food shops (and not the snack and supplement pumping chains), organic farm shops, markets, local food links projects and farmers markets, organic box schemes, fruit and veg wholesalers, and so on. Leave behind the supermarket trolley, the ghastly packaging filled aisles, and the zombifying checkout queues!

As part of a package of lifestyle changes, significantly increase the proportion of raw fruit and veg that you eat, IN AN INFORMED WAY – this will help create a more equitable and compassionate world, with much healthier and therefore probably happier and more fulfilled human beings.

The problem IS the solution, and working with nature is the way to naturally vibrant health.

Imagine the impacts when at least 5% to 10% of the population is eating at least 50% raw and more than 1% of the population is on at least a two-thirds raw diet – all at least partially supplied by organic forest gardening and agro-forestry. Think of the benefits in health, and then imagine the knock-on effects for the health service, in agriculture and the food supply industry. It is worth sitting for a few minutes, perhaps with your eyes closed, and imagining this future... and your part in it...

It could just start a peaceful and positive, healthy revolution... And with about 10% of the population vegetarian in Britain now, if at least half of vegetarians ate 50% raw or more then you can understand that this positive and healthy revolution could be started quite easily.

The Many Benefits: Multi-Function and Multi-Supply

So what is the role of permaculture in all this? Permaculture considers how one thing is placed in relation to others – such as the house and the parts of the garden where you grow your food. This is the idea of *relative location* – the location and conscious placement of one thing relative to many others. So in permaculture you grow your salads, soft-fruit and herbs close to the house (not at the end of the garden) because this uses less of your energy, gives the important 'used-every-day' part of the garden lots of attention because you can see it all very easily, and therefore makes it more productive.

Permaculture also aims to make sure that each part of a system has its needs met from a number of sources of supply, as well as providing a number of uses or benefits itself – *multi-function* and *multi-supply*. An example is a 'fedge'. This is a food producing hedge (fruits, as well as hedge-row salad plants such as hedge garlic), that can also be a boundary, a mulch producer and a sun-trap/wind break providing shelter to other food plants, as well as a wildlife habitat, a teacher and a thing of beauty.

Permaculture aims to mimic nature by creating a multi-layered 'forest garden' – this is *stacking* which is explained in more detail a little later. A forest garden is a wonderful example of multi-function and multi-supply. By carefully designing and growing a wide diversity of food plants together you create a wide range of supplies of food, as well as creating a food growing system that also protects and improves soil and water resources, that creates an excellent habitat for wildlife, and which creates an ecosystem that largely manages itself, with plants, insects and other wildlife all working together to meet each others needs from their natural outputs. So for example falling leaves and dead annual plants create a good mulch layer which becomes humus, which enriches the soil and then feeds the plants again, which then drop their leaves... so a natural cycle that builds fertility is established and maintained.

Permaculture always considers the 'ripple effects' of actions throughout the web of connections between elements in a system, the web of life and of aspects of our lifestyle – such as where or who we get our food from, and who gets the profit from what we buy. And that is one of the main roles of permaculture; to help us produce more of our own high quality, highly nutritious, fresh organic food, either personally, locally or bio-regionally.

Using simple ideas, a well designed diet with a high proportion of raw foods can serve several functions as well as producing numerous benefits – for example:

An Ecological Function: 'Greening' my life. Benefits: producing and eating more raw plant foods reduces resource and energy use, and promotes organics through higher food awareness. It significantly reduces demand for land, water and energy-hungry arable and animal farming. It promotes wildlife because it creates greater landscape diversity, normally means eating more tree crops (i.e. fruit) and reduces the overall need for agricultural land.

A Compassionate Function: A 'cruelty free' life. Benefits: a natural, mainly raw, vegan diet minimises animal exploitation and suffering, and reduces human suffering by promoting health, rather than creating illness.

An Economic Function: Producing and eating affordable, good quality, healthy, organic food and more positively directed spending. Benefits: a raw food diet can cut your food costs considerably, particularly if you get into permaculture and indoor sprouting. It can cut your energy costs and massively reduce health care costs. It can be used to avoid supporting the massive economic exploitation of the unsustainable global food production industry, which is dominated by just three hugely powerful companies: Nestlé, Unilever and Philip Morris Companies Inc. (see The Food System[38]). A significant change to healthier eating, as part of a holistic health strategy, will significantly reduce the huge long term health care costs that society will *have to* pay for i.e. you the tax payer, you the one that has to pay for expensive health insurance or treatment, etc. We can use our consumer power to promote positive, creative, healthy change towards sustainability. Invest in health creation, don't just pay up for insurance against illness!

[38] *The Food System*, by Tansey and Worsley (Earthscan, 1995), is an excellent book on the global food industry – reviewed in *Permaculture Magazine* Issue No. 11.

A Physical, Mental and Spiritual Health Function: Improving my health and vitality, in the short and long term. Benefits: a well designed natural diet promotes optimum health on all levels.

Some of the other simple benefits that I have experienced are:

❋ More vital, vibrant health: I feel more alive, with more energy.

❋ Improved sense of taste and smell, and generally more sensitivity – the food tastes great.

❋ Clearer head and more awake.

❋ Much less packaging and waste: no tin or aluminium cans, etc.

❋ Much less kitchen clutter – very few jars, bottles, packets, etc.

❋ Less use of energy: no need for freezer, fridge or cooker.

❋ Excellent clear and healthy skin, with little or no B.O. (a sweet smelling body in fact), reduced need for soaps, shampoos and less smelly clothes!

❋ A better understanding of one's body – and a more positive view of one's bodily functions!

Eating more raw foods can also be an easy and healthy way to lose a few unhealthy pounds (weight that is!). You can eat as much delicious raw foods as you want and if you are over-weight you will still lose pounds, and feel much better as a result. And for anyone worried about fitness, you should read Dr Douglas Graham's books or visit his website, see Appendix 3, if you really want to learn about superior health, fitness and strength that is achievable with a raw food lifestyle, or Stephen Arlin's book *Raw Power* on raw body building. In the UK there is a judo expert, who when he last competed in his 40's was still beating men ten years his junior, and a young canoeist, who was also competing in the top leagues. All over the world there are very many raw foodists who are very fit men and women who run, walk, cycle, dance, do lots of yoga...

Some 'Frequently Asked Questions' About Raw Foods
The Cooking Question

The first question is the cooking question: "so what's so bad about cooking if everyone's doing it?"

It's not really about attacking cooking, because cooking has come about for understandable reasons. Science accepts that physiologically and anatomically we are basically great apes – which means that even those of us that grew up in deepest darkest English commuter belt in Surrey (like I did) are tropical primates in biological terms. Since our emergence in the tropics we have spread to harsher northern climates where we eat and rely on many tougher foods that we did not evolve to eat, and which are not suited to being eaten raw by humans. The northern ecosystems offer less naturally digestible plant foods because there is less of the sun's energy to grow and ripen things. So to survive in an unnatural environment we had to cook loads of things to make them edible – to turn them from 'things' to 'food'. This enabled us to survive; so it's not about saying the past was 'wrong'. Instead it is about looking at where we are now, understanding the health and ecological effects of our foods, and then choosing where we want to head in the present and future. We can survive with these foods, but we cannot reach our true health potential, in this generation or in future generations.

Permaculture is about working with nature, and, put bluntly, as far as I can tell cooking (i.e. heating to a temperature that kills any life) does not play a part in any natural systems of life or ecology. Nature doesn't cook her foods for any creature; not one.

Did you know that the hotter you heat fat or oil the more toxic it becomes?

Nature is about life – cooked food is not biological; it has lost its life force. This might seem an extreme point of view – in fact it is a simple statement of the way things are. So despite what I thought a few years ago I now know that I do not need to cook food to live and thrive. I know from experience that I am both happier and healthier on a high percentage raw diet, and that it feels really good. I also know that permaculture can help us find much more ecological and efficient ways to feed ourselves in all climates; ways that are healthy and sustainable for both people and planet.

So if you are not convinced of the benefits of going 100% raw that's fine; I am sure you can sense however that there can only be benefits to yourself and the planet from eating more raw foods and particularly eating at least 50% raw plant foods.

The Protein Question

"So where do you get your protein from then?"

Well, take a look at the strength of any passing gorilla that happens to be strolling by, and ask it where it gets its protein from. Gorillas are the strongest primates, and they eat mainly leaves (about 95%) and just a little fruit – what's more they are pretty laid back too. A gorilla could quite easily rip your arm off – although it's not very likely to. So where does it get its strength from? Great apes thrive naturally on a low protein diet; that's what they are designed for – yet they are still incredibly strong.

How much protein do humans actually need? Can nature give us any clues? Well, human breast milk has no more than 2% to 3% protein, which is very low in comparison with many other animals, and that's at the time in life when we need more protein to build our growing baby bodies with. It is a perfectly designed natural food. It tells us a lot about our protein needs.

In humans the growth of osteoporosis, especially amongst high concentrated protein users such as athletes, is now suggesting that a high protein diet is in fact positively unhealthy. This seems to be because protein has to be broken down by the body to be passed through – it cannot pass through the body undigested. A high protein diet creates an acid body because of the more acidic digestive juices that are needed to break down protein. Carnivore's digestive juices are about 10 times more acid than our own, so that they can break down meat and get it out of their system fast, before it putrefies badly.

When we eat a lot of protein and our body becomes acid, the body then has to draw minerals from its own stored mineral reserves if it is to balance the body's pH; and it has to balance the body's pH, because if the blood goes out of a very narrow neutral to slightly alkaline range we die. So processing all this protein puts a lot of stress on the body. And because it is not getting the minerals it needs in a normal cooked and processed diet, the only place it can get minerals from is our body's stores – particularly our bones. Hence the depletion of calcium in the bones linked with osteoporosis. Research also shows that cultures and tribes that tend to live longer often have a low protein diet. In cases such as the Hunza Indians living to 120 to 130 years old has been common place... based on a low protein diet.

All the 'beasts of burden' used by man derive their great strength from an herbivorous, low protein diet. So what is it that builds a horse's power and a gorilla's strength? It's the essential amino-acids because they are what allow the body to build proteins itself, and therefore the muscles, and the same goes for the human body. We can get all the protein and protein building materials we need from vegetables in particular and fruit – green leafy vegetables, believe it or not, are the real wonders. And if you want to look into this question much more, you will find all the answers you need and more in Dr Douglas Graham's books, as well as the Nature's First Law books, *The Sunfood Diet Success System* (by David Wolfe) and *Raw Power* (by Stephen Arlin); the latter book being about raw food body building.

The Fat Question

There are various opinions amongst raw food advocates on the issue of fats, what fats are good and bad, and how much of them we should be eating. Recently some clearer, more helpful views have been expressed on this issue. Dr Douglas Graham and Fred Paténaude are amongst those that believe that being careful not to eat too many fats is important – very important even. On the other hand, at his talks I have heard David Wolfe say things like 'you can never eat too many avocados', whilst also stating that pure coconut oil is a fabulous food.

Personally, I think fats *are* important foods. And I find David Wolfe's argument interesting – which is that good quality fats are needed to dissolve the fats that contain poisons which are stored in our body, because water (including the water of fruits) cannot dissolve or break down fats. However, my personal experience is that I have always felt at my best, my lightest, and most energetic when I have had a low proportion of raw vegetable fats in my diet (from avocados, oils, nuts and / or seeds). From what I have observed in myself and others, excessive eating of fats is often linked to serious over-eating, often covering up emotional issues. And I have also seen that those that eat a low fat diet generally come over as more balanced and in control of their lives, emotions and energies in a relaxed and healthy way.

I sense that our natural, 'evolutionary' diet would have quite possibly included a slightly higher proportion of fats than our closest genetic relatives because we have a bigger brain – and our brain is basically a big lump of rather complex and amazing fatty tissue, for which vegetable fatty acids are the ideal building and maintenance materials. But I do not believe we would have eaten a lot of fats, except on odd occasions. The fats would have always been in a natural, whole state, combined in the fruit or food that they were part of. Processed foods, even if they are cold pressed virgin oils, are still processed foods – they are not whole foods, designed by nature. Processing of any form involves extra energy, packaging and transport, and changes the food from its natural and therefore healthiest form. Often it is just another case of someone wanting to sell you something to 'make a living'.

Douglas Graham's new booklet *Fruit or Fat?* will be essential reading for anyone interested in the detail of these issues. The standard American diet (SAD) obtains 42% of its calories from its fat intake, and this is about the same for vegans and vegetarians. He points out that often without realising it raw fooders can be eating up to 80% fat in their diet by calories! This is particularly likely for those that eat a lot of avocados, and / or nuts, seeds and oils – which can easily happen for those eating more salads than fruits.

Some key points that Dr Graham highlights are that fats, whether cooked or raw, clog up the cardiovascular system, and reduce the oxygen carrying capacity of the blood, which adversely affects cell functioning, and therefore for example can lead to reduced clarity of thinking. Another key point is that to deal with the excessive fats the body releases more adrenaline to drive the pancreas to produce the higher levels of insulin that the body needs to deal with the fats in the bloodstream. This can lead to adrenal exhaustion and pancreatic fatigue. So blood sugar levels can be all over the place, and this can then cause general chronic fatigue, as well as hyper and hypo-glycemia, candida, diabetes and other serious conditions.

Dr Graham cites the recommendations of the Pritkin Longevity Center, which he says has 'the finest health-regeneration record of any organisation in the US'. They recommend no more than 10% fat in your diet, and using this as a base Doug Graham states that 80/10/10 is the target for optimum health – 80% of calories from simple carbohydrates (from fruit sugars), with 10% fat and 10% protein. This he says is 'by far the most healthful and sustainable raw-food approach'.

Certainly Douglas Graham and the professional athletes and sports people he advises are evidence in themselves that you can enjoy an extremely high level of fitness on a low fat, low protein, high fruit, raw diet.

The Meat Question

"So what about chimpanzees eating meat then?"

Yes, we humans can and do eat meat. Does this mean it is good for our mind-body-spirit system and the planetary system to do so? We can smoke cigarettes, drive our cars hundreds of miles day-in day-out, unwittingly become victims to alcoholism, we can even use heroin and abuse and murder each other but that does not mean these are good things for us. These are health and lifestyle choices that affect our own body and the planet as a whole. All I can say is that I feel better in my mind, body and spirit not eating meat.

I am not into meat-eater bashing. Most of my life I have been a meat eater – I changed in my mid twenties. This was linked to my walks in the beautiful Hampshire countryside where I regularly came across hidden battery chicken houses, with their grey atmosphere of death and disease; then seeing lorries passing through Alton and Petersfield town centres crammed with thousands of boxed-in chickens, on their way to the slaughterhouse; and then not being able to find a chicken in the supermarket with a straight spine or unbroken legs – I started to make the links.

I can only speak from personal experience and I know that the reasons for my lifestyle changes have combined logical reasoning, based on sound information from people and sources that I trust, alongside a strong sense of what feels like the right thing for me and what I want to do.

As for the commonplace retort 'but chimpanzees eat meat'. Yes, indeed some of them do, yet they do so only occasionally. And consider for a moment the behaviour associated with their meat eating. Chimpanzee's meat eating is usually part of a kind of frenzied and barbaric, territorial slaughter; some of it even cannibalistic. We have a different moral, ethical and contemplative capacity to chimpanzees. We can consider and digest more information, both rational and ethical, and in doing so we make decisions. Some humans kill people; it doesn't mean I should. The Olympic athletes of ancient Greece ate mainly fruit; their soldiers on the other hand were fed meat.

We have much, much smaller canine teeth than chimps. And whilst we share 98.4% of our genes with chimpanzees, I've been told that we also share about 60% of our genes with bananas!

Suggesting that we need to eat meat because chimpanzees have been found to eat meat is a rather bizarre form of logic. However, let's follow it through. Even at its base level it implies we should ALWAYS eat our meat fresh and raw, and we should always go out and kill it ourselves – by hand. It also suggests we should eat meat far less often than we do... and that we should eat at least 95% fresh, ripe, raw fruit and leaves as chimpanzees do... with some nice juicy insects and grubs, and a tiny amount of raw meat. How do you fancy that then? If you want to follow that argument then logic is plain and simple.

Do humans tend to prefer the smell of a fruit 'n' veg warehouse or a slaughter house? If this logic is being used then the essentially fruitarian habits of Orangutans and Bonobos, and the mainly leaf-eating habits of Gorillas are equally relevant. And if you are really into the 'what about chimpanzees eating meat?' thing you will find that our closest genetic/DNA relative is actually the Bonobo or Pygmy Chimpanzee. These are more placid and more intelligent than their heavier relatives, only occasionally eating insects and eggs. They live in close and affectionate groups, using sexual interaction rather than violence when they feel stress, and they also have a matriarchal society. Make of that what you will.

Yes, we are incredibly adaptable, so yes we can eat meat but it is increasingly obvious that our high meat consumption is both a narrow socio-cultural norm and a physical and economic addiction that is generating significant costs in terms of human and environmental health.

The Starch Question

"But what about starch then?"

The body needs sugars (simple carbohydrates) as its fuels, yes, but it does not need starches (complex carbohydrates). Starches are turned into more easily digested sugars, and it actually involves a lot more work for the body to break the starches down into the sugars it needs in comparison with taking those sugars directly from fruit. Again look to our closest relatives, our anatomy and physiology, and our digestive system. Look to what we are naturally designed to eat, not what we eat habitually. We are very clearly not designed by nature to eat grains or grain products[39].

Highly processed starches are actually a major problem for the body to digest and clog up the digestive system a great deal, especially when combined with cooked fats. They are one of the main components of the 'rubber tar' that lines your digestive system if you are on a normal diet, which prevents the proper assimilation of nutrients, reduces our capacity to digest food, and which is known as mucoid plaque.

The Nutritional Research Question

It is interesting to look at things the other way around, and be aware of what happens when chimpanzees are fed a conventional human diet. In research, this leads to serious illness in the chimpanzees and all sorts of behavioural problems. What does that suggest?

Research at Exeter University by ex-police officer Peter Bennett found that a diet with a high proportion of raw fruit and veg significantly helped in reducing behavioural problems, such as stress and aggressiveness, in young offenders and young soldiers. Mineral and vitamin balances were the key. [40]

---

[39] See Dr Douglas Graham's excellent booklet *Grain Damage* for more detailed information on the subject of grains.

[40] *Writings on Nutrition and Behaviour*, Peter Bennett, Gail Bradley and Nicholas Bennett (Behavioural Health Partnership).

The problem with nutritional research is not that it comes up with 'wrong' answers but that its starting point and questions are based on hidden assumptions i.e. cooked food is the base line because that's what is normal in our society, and what is normal for a nutrition researcher. It is not starting with a clean sheet. It's asking the wrong questions.

In fact, if you look into it there is often more genuine, objective science in primate nutrition in zoos and primate research than there is science in the field of human nutrition because it is actually based on anatomy and physiology, while the 'science' of human nutrition is not. Given the sophistication of our knowledge in certain areas, if we were truly scientific in our study of human health and nutrition we would quite obviously all be healthy by now. Think about it.

Science and research is often largely driven by the private sector undertaking its own research, or funding university research on topics the funders select. Drug companies inevitably fund research that involves drugs; they are not going to fund research, however positive it might be, that suggests we would need few (if any) of the drugs they produce if we followed a different, more natural route. There is not much profit (at the moment) in creating a healthy population.

As an example of this, a TV programme on the links between diet and brain degeneration detailed a long term and very rigorous study of thousands of people in the USA, which suggested that meat eaters were 2 to 3 times more likely to suffer from dementia than vegetarians. Despite the huge implications for human health, the researchers were unable to gain funding support to take their studies further.

Patterns of thinking tend to be the same in most academic and research areas. 'Reductionism'[41] leads to the kind of internal consistency that allow economists, genetic engineers, agro-chemists and politicians to justify their actions within their own intellectually clever but inevitably narrow perspectives, when often their arguments just don't make sense when considered within a wider view. So the patterns of thinking that developed modern nutritional science are exactly the same as those that developed GMOs, toxic agro-chemicals and lots, and lots, and lots of pharmaceutical drugs. Nutritional science contains a lot of useful information and many powerful ideas, but that doesn't mean that nutritional science has got it all 'right'. Drug research starts from a solid belief in drugs; and virtually all nutritional research starts with a solid belief in cooked foods.

A key fact to understand is that nutritional research is not based on our anatomy, biology or physiology. It has been developed by looking at the nutritional contents of what we normally eat (i.e. what foods are marketed to us) in our western culture.

Nutrition research, like the vast majority of research, has also got to the

---

[41] Looking narrowly at a subject, and ignoring its wider context and connections with other topics.

point where it is totally focused on the minutiae of its subject. It has many assumptions (for example, in relation to proteins and carbohydrates), which became firmly established at a time when research was far less sophisticated... and those assumptions are largely forgotten or ignored. If nutritional research started now with a clean sheet of paper then I think it would get the right answers quite quickly. But it is starting with a sheet of paper full of old ideas, and therefore it is asking the wrong kinds of questions.

For example, as Loren Lockman points out: *"It's important to understand that it's not what nutrients are in the food that's most important, but rather, what nutrients the body is able to easily assimilate."*[42] Modern nutrition is gradually shifting in a positive direction, but it is still largely food based, focusing on the theoretical nutritional content of the food. It ignores physiological science, which is much better at identifying what nutrients our body is able to assimilate most easily. So nutritional researchers still aren't really seeing the wood for the trees. They are understandably studying the nutrients that are in the normal western diet, but we all know already that that diet is well suited to creating illness and disease. There are many fewer nutritionists that are actually studying the nutrition that creates vibrant health. So if you want to be vibrantly health you have to look carefully at where your nutritional advice is coming from – is it health creating nutrition, or 'normal' nutrition?

How many nutritional researchers have actually done any research on high percentage or totally raw foods diets? How many nutritionists are basing their opinions about raw food on extensive research into raw foods, or on any knowledge and experience of people following a raw food lifestyle? Or how many researchers have any long term experience of eating a significant proportion of raw foods themselves? This is the best possible form of research and it is of course the one that raw foodists follow!

There are those listed early in Part One of this book. But there is virtually no current funded institutional research, except for some work at Cornell University in the US and one study at Geissen University in Germany a few years ago that I know of – which came up with very clear positive results but which was unable to gain funding to take the research further and properly promote the results. So most nutritionists will come out with uninformed statements about raw food diets, based on no knowledge or research of the subject. This is hardly surprising as it challenges all their basic assumptions, as well as their expert reputations and therefore their livelihoods, and their own diets.

If you start looking at accepted research in other areas, such as anatomy and physiology what do we find? We find plenty of scientifically accepted facts that contradict the conventional nutritional perspective. We find through simple observation of nature that animals are basically totally and vibrantly healthy. And these perspectives tells us that all forms of life have a specific physiology, which is ideally

[42] *A Handbook for Vibrant Living – Eight Keys to Optimal Health*, Loren Lockman, Natural Designs Publishing (2001), 5825 Tanglewood Drive, Bethesda, MD 20817, USA. www.TanglewoodWelln essCenter.com

suited for a specific diet. What this suggests is that if you choose for yourself total, vibrant health then there is only one place to be – and that's working with nature.

'Okham's Razor' is a famous philosophical and scientific tool, which states that given all other things being equal the simplest explanation will be true. So if we are looking at the human anatomy and physiology, the simplest explanation for it being as it is will be that, like every other form of life, it is perfectly designed by nature to eat a particular type of food. So our human anatomy and physiology tells us what nature's perfect food for us is. Lockman points out that 'God', 'Goddess', universe, nature, creation, evolution did not screw it up – they provided us with all we need for natural health.

So if two animals share the same basic physiology they share the same natural diet/optimum nutrition. Our body is designed to eat foods, which are 80% water. Primates typically don't drink a lot, because their foods are so full of water. All animals sharing human physiology eat primarily fruit, with at most 25% leaves and 2-3% protein in their diet. Gorillas, with larger stomachs and slightly different physiology eat mainly leaves (although they prefer fruit if it is available). Bonobos always eat only fruit whenever they can. In nature all animals keep their meals simple. Which suggests that it is most natural, and therefore most healthy to eat simple meals.

I and many others have removed our unspoken assumptions about food. From years of experience I know that it feels far 'better' to my mind-body-spirit, and 'better' for my relationship with the earth as a whole, if I eat a high proportion of raw foods. 'Better' means I feel more at ease living in this way – healthier and happier – my mind is more content and my body feels better, and the ripple effects feel more positive.

On a purely logical level, I know that I do not need to eat cooked food, meat or dairy produce, so I do not. I also recognise now that the dairy and meat industries are one-and-the-same, and they influence the pattern of arable farming enormously because of their huge demand for land for growing feedstuffs. In ecological terms, industrialised animal farming is highly inefficient, using as it does vast quantities of water and agro-chemicals – which means big incomes for the agro-chemical giants. Dairy produce and the gluten in wheat is very 'mucus forming', which means it clogs up the body and hampers the efficiency of the immune system. And to grow wheat we mimic its natural habitat – we create semi-desert to feed our wheat habit; and a 'habit' it is because wheat includes addictive chemicals of the opiate family.[43]

So, whether you stop or just cut down significantly, reducing the amount of meat, dairy and wheat products that you eat will have many benefits. Some of these might not be obvious, so it might help to sit quietly for a moment and imagine some of the knock-on effects...

Despite what people who are new to the idea of raw food lifestyles often

---

[43] See the booklet *Grain Damage* by Dr Douglas Graham, which can be obtained from the FRESH Network, Living Nutrition, Nature's First Law, etc.

expect, it just feels natural. And because it is working with nature I find it an easier way of life, that is not a struggle or an effort. There's no greasy washing up or tough pan cleaning either!

Some suggestions for you if you want to take time to consider the issues:

✳ Understand the nature and effects of foods that are heavy and slow, that take a lot of energy to digest and that therefore make us feel sleepy as we don't have enough energy to digest them and stay awake at the same time. To blast away this sleepiness we habitually use five main stimulants: caffeine, sugar, nicotine, salt and protein.

✳ Get to know the foods that are cleansing, life giving and energising. Get a feel in your body for the biology and bio-chemistry of foods.

✳ Study the science of life and evolution. By this I do not mean studying scientific ideas about life and evolution (although some of it is obviously extremely useful). What I mean is using your own observation and experience to get a really deep feel for the foods and growing systems that increase life energy; and get in touch with your body's 'innate intelligence'. Taste the foods you eat fully – and listen to your body; allow it to tell you which foods feel like they will create health.

The practicalities of this lifestyle, such as transitional living, all year salad beds, perennial vegetables, forest gardening, sprouting and the plants for a future concept, are dealt with in the next section of this book.

AVOCADOS

PART 2
The Practicalities

Transitional Living

There are different routes to changing your life. You can just stop what you are doing and change your life completely – it is possible. Some people do just stop smoking cigarettes, or drinking alcohol or coffee for example – all of which are addictive drugs.

The same can happen when making wholesale changes in one's diet. And if you do suddenly start eating all raw or nearly all raw the first one or two weeks can be difficult – particularly the first 2 to 4 days, because this is when the body starts to clean itself out. But after that you will feel so much better.

Some suggest that a slow transition can make it much more difficult to take the final step, and that a clear and determined change is best. If someone is trying to stop smoking for example, slowly cutting down from 40-a-day to one or two cigarettes per day is a big change – but it is still very, very different to giving up completely. And not giving up completely prevents the really significant changes from happening.

Others say that a slow transition is much better. This allows a more gentle release of the toxins in the body and therefore controls the physical and emotional reactions to the detoxification process – although the benefits of this approach depend on what you are eating. The cooked proportion of your diet needs to be relatively healthy too. If you are still eating 50% junk food or highly processed food, grains, meat or dairy you are still not eating a good enough diet to get anything important cleaned out of your system. So it's a question of choosing what you feel will work for you. The most important thing is your state of mind and emotions – how you feel about making the change. If you feel clear, and positive or determined then it will be easier. If you think you should change but don't really want to it won't be so easy.

With raw food a clear and rapid change to eating mainly raw fruits and vegetables is not a problem. I recommend it completely. A change to eating 100% raw is very different though to eating mainly raw. For a lot of people it is quite a challenge to go 100% and stick to it, although some do manage it with no great problems. For most people a transition period is what happens whether they want to or not. During this time they are eating a lot more raw food, but not 100%, some deliberately, and some because they have a bit of 'slippage' and give into some of the cravings for cooked food that often come up. A planned transition to 70-90% raw is very practical, and then move on to 100% if you want to, when you want to. The main thing is to feel good about what you are doing, and if you do have 'slippage' understand that it is perfectly OK – you are moving in the right direction, and giving your body more and more of an opportunity to create health.

Overall, giving up processed food is by far the most important first step. Do this and it will make a big difference to your health; especially processed fats, and processed carbohydrates (yes, that includes wheat products) and sugars. Basically, the message is 'get off processed foods as fast as you can' – because that is the stuff that really messes with nature. It is chemically totally different to anything natural. Putting it in our bodies inevitably has a big effect on both our mind and emotions, as well as our body. Think it through. And then think through the effects from one generation to the next, recognising that we have only really had one full generation of highly processed food eating so far.

Dr Udo Erasmus in his excellent book and tapes *'Fats That Kill, Fats That Heal'* states that there are five 'killer fats'. These are basically the highly processed and cooked fats, such as the highly processed fats used in margarines – and it is quite shocking to discover the processes that these fats typically go through to make margarine. So for anyone on a 'normal' diet one of the best first steps is to get off cooked and highly processed fats. Dr Erasmus then goes on to explain how Omega 3 and Omega 6 fats are particularly valuable and have tremendous healing properties.

When you do get right off processed foods you will be amazed and delighted at the results within two to three weeks.

Cut right down or preferably cut out these things and at the same time add in more raw nutrition. A raw fruit breakfast, and just fruit in the morning, with more green salad vegetables as part of later meals is often the best way to go initially. Going straight to a high fruit diet can make some people feel a bit 'spacey' because they are not used to it. Fruit is also more cleansing and will lead to toxins being released into the blood. Brief dizzy spells when you stand up might happen when you come off coffee or junk food, for example – be aware of this but don't worry about it, it's just the body getting stuff out through the blood stream and adjusting its chemical balances. If you go for mainly fruit, over time the high energy that will result from it may need some grounding through meditation, yoga, or eating more greens. In the garden or your window boxes start with an all-year salad garden planted up over a series of weekends, and try some sprouting indoors.

In discovering either permaculture or raw food (or both), often when people find out about these things, they think 'oh, I must do this right'. However, it is really important that you don't give yourself a hard time for not being as 'perfect' as you think you should be or for feeling it is hard to make changes in your life. Food is a very important part of peoples' lives whether they realise it or not. Making major changes can be challenging... as well as amazingly liberating.

If you gradually just eat more healthy raw fruits and vegetables you can't make many mistakes, although you can make a few – which this book will help you avoid. Frederic Paténaude's book *Raw Secrets*, is also very good for being open, honest and direct about some potential raw food pitfalls.

You and your body will be learning as you go. The same goes for planting and growing your own foods, and developing permaculture in your life. Both these changes in your lifestyle offer long term opportunities to learn and experiment.

Getting started and just having a go, even doing this playfully, is the most important thing. The main thing is to feel that you are heading in the right direction, which involves gaining better information to start with. You don't have to do it overnight – you don't have to switch from cooked food one day to eating 100% raw the next day. And you don't have to create the 'perfect' forest garden in a weekend either! Start by reducing or cutting out processed foods, while increasing the proportion of raw food you include in your diet, and see what benefits accrue. The benefits of these changes in your life may take a little time to become clear, and will depend on what type and proportion of raw and home grown foods you include in your diet.

When you increase the amount of fruit and raw foods you eat there are a few things that are really useful to know about:

* Ideally, eat fruit on its own and eat it before your meal rather than after, because it is digested quickly and easily (about half an hour if it is ripe). This avoids fruit combining with starches or concentrated proteins which can set up a ferment (i.e. wind/gas!). Apples are a bit of an exception, as they combine well with leaf and vegetable salads. Simple, fruit-only breakfasts/mornings are a great way to start the day.

* Develop an understanding of food combining. When you taste food this sends signals to the stomach about what type of food it is. Starches and proteins require different types of digestive juices for best digestion. Combining starches and proteins, or starches and sugars creates fermentation in the digestive system, which prevents digestion. Mixing green and non-starchy vegetables with protein foods or starches is a good combination. The nitty-gritty of this is that there are three bacterial processes that can happen in the digestive system – two are bad and one is good. They are digestion, fermentation and putrefaction. Digestion is the good process whereby we assimilate nutrition, which is in fact the excretions of good bacteria (lacto-bacteria) in the digestive system. Fermentation (of starches) and putrefaction (of proteins) happen when unhealthy and badly combined foods are eaten, which are then broken down by the bacteria in the digestive system but in these cases producing toxic excretions.

* Another useful tip is always to start your main meal with something raw like salad, ideally without any dressing, at least for the first few mouthfuls, or if you do use a dressing use cold pressed oils because they are untreated; and freshly squeezed lemon juice. The body then thinks the whole meal will be raw and avoids digestive leucocytosis, leaving the immune system more able to deal with anything that it needs to tackle.

✳ An important point is that your nutritional health depends on your body's ability to assimilate that nutrition. If your digestive system is caked with undigested starches, cooked fats and other food debris – as most people's are – then it is difficult for the nutrition in the food to make its way through that 'gack'. So eating the best foods is far, far better than eating the worst foods – but to get the most out of those good foods you also need to take some actions to clean up your digestive system, and fortunately the best raw plant foods will help you do that. Then you will really feel the benefits most. So the first part of your transition is a cleansing process, and that is something you can design or manage. Just having fresh fruit juice for several days – 'a juice fast' – is a very good way to accelerate this, and normally people really enjoy it. Fully cleansing out the system actually needs more radical action like herbal cleanses, longer fasts or colonics because of the mucoid plaque that was mentioned earlier – it is not natural for it to be there, so the body does not have a natural mechanism to get rid of it. It's tough stuff to shift![44]

✳ Try to make sure you don't become paranoid and obsessed about raw food or food in general, thinking you have to 'get it right' all the time, and thinking or feeling you have to be a 'perfect' raw fooder or fruitarian. What you are doing is making positive changes; improving the chain of cause-and-effect within your body and in the wider world. Food is not everything in life, by any means!

Making the Transition

Dr Joel Robbins suggests that a good way to make a gradual change in diet is not to cut all the foods you like out of your diet but simply to add more raw foods in. Gradually as you eat a higher proportion of raw foods your body will guide you in a way that feels good. You will often then be drawn to eat more raw foods by what Dr Robbins calls the body's 'innate intelligence'. In this way Dr Robbins even found that his fanatical enjoyment of hot and spicy Mexican food disappeared without any loss of pleasure or satisfaction from his food. He continued to eat the occasional Mexican meal when he wanted, when otherwise he was fully raw.[45] Frederic Paténaude on the other hand emphasises that all bad habits are bad habits, and smaller bad habits will still prevent you getting healthy, and will remain a cause of sickness and disease.

In the best selling book *Raw Energy* Leslie and Susannah Kenton suggest another good gradual transition is to have an 'apple day' once a week, where you just have apples for breakfast and lunch initially. And then apples for every meal one day per week when you feel like it. Apples are excellent foods for such an approach because they are so well balanced in vitamins and minerals.

---

[44] For more information on this you can explore any number of raw food books or visit the Karuna Retreats website – www.karunaretreats.com

[45] And for those that love hot and spicy foods, check out 'Chris's Amazing Raw Curry' on page 146.

Putting too much pressure on yourself and others can make the journey more difficult, and less fun. It can be worth taking things slowly at first if that makes it more likely that you get to where you really want to be – although it is important to have a clear goal. For example you might like to set some monthly targets for yourself. Some people prefer to make more rapid changes. If this is well informed, it will bring the benefits of change more quickly, although it may also intensify the symptoms in any cleansing process. A more rapid approach means you will have the objective of getting these out of the way more quickly and this can work for those that enjoy the possibility of a challenge – physical, mental, emotional and/or spiritual.

The first most obvious transition is to just have fresh fruit for breakfast. This can also immediately demonstrate the great time and energy saving benefits of raw eating. I started (in autumn going into winter of all times) by switching to an all fruit breakfast and having a salad, with home-sprouted organic seeds or pulses for lunch. In the evening I had another salad, and added steamed potatoes or lightly cooked millet half way through. It is worth pointing out that salad to me does not mean lettuce, cucumber and tomato; it means something much more interesting and enjoyable than that! I quickly found that it doesn't take much effort to experiment and learn the huge and delicious variety of things you can use to create a salad – especially if you grow a little rocket, oriental saladini and herbs for yourself. Without me really noticing, my body's desire for the starchy foods disappeared during the winter, and when Spring arrived I found it much easier and enjoyable to grab a bag of apples for lunch than to make a salad. When this happened I found that without making a decision to do so I had switched from two thirds salad and one third fruit to one third salad and two thirds fruit – which felt both natural and great!

Many raw educators, with Professor Arnold Ehret being one of the most well known and respected, emphasise that foods don't cure anything at all. The body itself cures everything. Every organism is self-healing, and perfect health is the normal and natural condition for a body. As Loren Lockman says: 'you just have to get out of the way. You just have to learn how to stop creating disease to allow the body to heal itself'. If we learn this individually, in our families and communities, and as a society then vitality, strength and superb health will be the natural result.

This practical, first-steps approach is important for permaculture, creating community and any other aspect of change towards a more ecological and humane way of life. The process of change itself must be sustainable – which means it needs to feel good to you. You may want to go on some workshops or courses, to contact networks and know where to find information and support from people you share common ideals and motivations with (see Appendix 3). Allow change to happen by recognising that the world and your life is a constant flow of change. Movement is always happening although at times it may seem slow – at other time it may feel like a roller-coaster ride!

We all have the ability to make choices and we base our choices on our experience and the information we have to hand. So there is no intention here of forcing anyone to change their diet – the choice is yours. However, I do humbly suggest that you base your choices on good information and on careful observation. Explore the subject; do your own research by having a go, and keep your eyes, your heart and your mind open while considering the important issues in your life. I hope that this book can help you in that process, and lead you towards a diet and a lifestyle that feels right for you.

Detox: - the body's natural detoxification process

'Detox' is something important to know about. It is a natural detoxification process that the body initiates when it has the opportunity (the energy and resources) to do so. This happens when your body has health creating foods coming in and therefore has the chance to clear out some of the 'rubbish' it has stored in it. It also happens when it has no food, and just water coming in – this is fasting. Detoxification can be rather like having a cold, because it's your body's opportunity to clear some gunk and mucous! Early on, a detox may also include some bowel clearance as your body flushes out stored toxins that it has decided it is now safe to release. If you know what's happening you can even welcome this, knowing that it is about your body doing what comes naturally and that means using it's innate intelligence to create health.

During a detox there are a range of symptoms that you might experience, such as:

* Fuzzy headedness or headaches: flushed out toxins in the blood affecting the brain.

* Clogged up, or a running nose: release of unwanted mucous.

* Sore throat: a sensitive area affected by toxins released into the blood.

* Mouth ulcers: release of toxins through the sensitive skin of the mouth.

* Weariness: toxins in the blood affecting the muscles.

* Itchy skin: toxins coming out through the skin, which is the largest organ of the body.

* Irritability: released toxins affecting how one feels and therefore moods.

* Unpleasant breath and body odours: toxins released through skin and breath.

These effects are some of the physical and emotional results of a bunch of rather nasty and unnatural chemicals (i.e. things you've eaten!) being released into the bloodstream and lymphatic system, which the body doesn't feel very comfortable about. Muscular weariness and lethargy can be caused when toxins come into the blood from where the body has been forced to store them (often fat cells). With toxins coming into the system the natural response of the body is to want to rest because it needs to divert energies away from its normal activities in order to cope with the extra work of processing and ridding itself of higher levels of toxins. So a feeling of weariness can result. It's the body telling you "rest me, so that I can direct my energy to dealing with this stuff I want to get rid of!" Plenty of sleep or dozing will usually help the detox because it will give the body a good period of rest from eating. And if you don't feel like eating don't eat, just drink water.

However, it's never quite that simple. Sometimes at the same time as these unpleasant effects there can be very positive feelings of exhilaration that result from the body's removal of toxins. Sometimes there can even be a strange mixture of weariness, as well as a strong desire to be active, to do physical exercise, run or do some sport or yoga. This is because activity helps to get the blood pumping and to improve the release of toxins through the lymphatic system and organs, including sweat through the skin.

Many people concerned with health, and not just raw fooders, understand that we have to go through this detox process if we want to strive for real health – because we have to shift from the body the toxins that pose a long term threat to our health. Fasting, saunas, sweat lodges, and herbal cleanses are other ways of stimulating the detox process. However, unless you're fairly well cleaned out already, it is not really advisable to combine all these together! The immune system is the driving force behind the detox and cleansing process. So all these techniques are just ways of strengthening, 'lubricating' or stimulating the immune system and its innate intelligence.

Have you noticed how so many children seem to have a constantly running nose or cough? This is natural in that the child's body is naturally trying to rid itself of the mucous it gets from dairy and wheat foods in particular, as well as the toxins that come into its body in any crisps, fried or highly processed foods. Most reasonably healthy children on a normal diet are in an almost constant state of detox with snotty noses. Those on the worst diets or who are over-weight are often not detoxing and don't get such bad colds because their body has too much to cope with already in 'just surviving' mode. This is quite obviously not because they are healthier. It is not necessarily easy helping children to establish a truly healthy diet, but fortunately there are now books, magazines and networks available to help. The main issue is that normally the child wants to copy the parent, particularly with younger children. So if the parent is happy and relaxed eating a lot of raw foods then so will the child be (more on this later).

If a detox is too rapid when someone has a lot of toxins stored in their body it is possible for it to have some dangerous effects. However, these are only possible if someone takes an extreme approach to detoxing, such as going straight into a one week water only fast straight from a junk food diet. Such an extreme approach can lead to a huge release of toxins into the blood if you've been eating a lot of junk. This can create an unnaturally high toxic overload which the body's organs and filters cannot cope with, and which can then pose some dangers, including to the brain. However, such effects will *not* normally occur even through fairly rapid and significant dietary changes. It would only happen if you go straight from a very toxic diet into a serious fast, which I would not recommend. Provided you are well informed, or have contact with others with knowledge and experience, and provided you maintain a good balance of vitamins and minerals, particularly fresh green vegetables, the benefits of detoxification greatly outweigh any short term unpleasant effects. There is no danger in a normal detox process, only benefits.

Detox is stimulated by eating more healthily, fasting or 'eating' just fresh juice, which then gives the body more energy and resources to clear out unwanted toxins. So detox symptoms can be stopped either by stopping the detox process itself by diverting energy and resources away from it, or by encouraging it to its natural conclusion. To encourage and assist it you should drink plenty of liquid, either spring water, fresh raw juices or distilled water to help flush the toxins through the body – carrot, beetroot, apple and celery based juices are really good for this. Well informed short fasts will also accelerate this cleansing process. Then using plenty of fresh greens is also important to help replenish the body, particularly if you are coming from a diet that has been very unhealthy. On the other hand, often going back to eating more normally (i.e. some cooked foods, such as steamed or lightly boiled vegetables) will normally stop the detox process where it is. The body's 'innate intelligence' will then take it up again when it feels ready – if you give it the chance.

Fasting is a particularly powerful route to cleansing and detoxification that has been and still is part of many, even most, spiritual traditions. This is because it creates challenges for mind, body and spirit in the fasting process which the faster can draw strength and understanding from overcoming, and also because it cleans and clears the mind, body and spirit allowing for a clearer and deeper spiritual connection in its latter stages and beyond.

It is essential to be well informed and well prepared before entering into a fast, because it can release a lot of stored toxins into the body very rapidly – which occasionally can be dangerous. The body needs to be in good shape to deal with the kind of cleansing a major fast can bring on. So do not go straight into serious fasting from a very poor diet (no more than 3 or 4 days) – read and consult others about it first, and make sure you've got others around you, or do a supervised fast. But a one to three day fast is not going to harm any one, and can only do good although it may well make you feel 'ill' because of the passage of toxins through the body in the process of getting them out. So if you try it just make sure you drink plenty of water to keep the body hydrated and to help flush the toxins through. Professor Arnold Ehret's superb book *Rational Fasting* is probably the best and most straight-forward there is on the subject, and has been a best seller for many years – it is also very cheap[46]. After curing himself of an 'incurable' disease through fasting, followed by many years of research into fasting, and perhaps unparalleled personal experience

---

[46] The FRESH Network supplies many books with excellent information on fasting; the tapes by Dr Joel Robbins are a superb source of information – everyone should listen to them!

for a westerner (including two scientifically supervised fasts of around 50 days) Professor Ehret recommended regular short fasts of perhaps three days to one week, but did not recommend the very long fasts which some more extreme people are drawn towards and which he undertook himself earlier in his life.

I do not have a lot of fasting experience... yet. But I have a lot of good friends that do. It is one area of my transition to raw foods that I would change looking back with hindsight, as I am only now starting to explore the benefits of sensible fasting. If I had known people with more fasting experience earlier on or read more on the subject earlier I am sure I would have done some short fasts soon into my transition to raw foods, and I know that this would have benefited me. Apart from the cleansing benefits I feel fasting also provides the body and emotions with confidence not to eat constantly. It helps break the unhealthy pattern of emotional eating and habitual eating that feeds an appetite that is used to eating far more than the body needs, at times when no nutrition is actually needed.

Generally, the aim of natural, healthy eating is to create a slightly alkaline body as this is the natural state for vibrant health. So your aim is to reduce the acid creating foods, and add in more alkaline foods. Many raw food books give guidance on what foods are most help in doing this. It is worth being aware that green leafs are by far the most alkaline of foods; melons, celery and cucumbers are also excellent alkalisers for the body. Nuts, grains and heavy protein foods are really the only raw foods you need to watch as they are more acid forming. Generally aiming for about 80% alkaline foods is a good guide. Dairy and meat, coffee and drugs (both medicines and recreational drugs) are some of the most extremely acidifying things our bodies have to cope with.

Trace minerals are important, and again this is where green leaves are particularly good – and where wild foods and perennial greens are best. Also it is worth knowing that some plants have particularly beneficial effects. For example, the vegetable fatty acids in avocados and plants such as *Ginkgo biloba*[47] are particularly good for the brain and neurological system because the brain and other organs are basically very sophisticated and important lumps of fat!

In his talks David Wolfe particularly emphasises the vital role of mineral rich foods because of the mineral depleted state of the soils our foods are grown in, and because minerals are needed to support the cleansing process. He stresses that green leafy vegetables are the very best sources of minerals, and some plants in particular are especially good providers of key minerals in their natural, organically bound form:

❋ Celery has some of the highest levels of natural, organically bound salts, and is therefore a very important food.

❋ Chromium is in cinnamon, magnesium is in saffron, and silicon, which

---

[47] Best in dried leaf form rather than in expensive processed tablets, harvested from the amazing Ginkgo tree – which can often be found in your local public park, once you know what this unique tree and its leaf looks like.

is a very important mineral, is found in very high levels in horsetail, nettles, hemp leaves and romaine lettuce. David Wolfe suggests that silicon is in fact a key mineral for healthy bones because it is required for the assimilation of other minerals including calcium – it is a catalyst required by the bone building process. Calcium is also very important for other things.

Gaining information or opinions on these trace nutrients is a choice. Personally, I'm a bit lazy in these matters and don't tend to worry about the specifics of exactly what minerals are in which foods – I just eat a good variety of fresh, home grown green vegetables, fruit and wild foods, confident from experience that the diversity and balance will give me what I need. This certainly gives me far more of the very best health building minerals, vitamins and enzymes than I ever had before I was raw.

All these factors can be part of your experience of change. You are always living in times of change; the one thing you can be sure of as constant, is perpetual change. Working with nature means working with change. Once accepted, this means you look towards making conscious changes in what you eat and how you obtain your food, and be happy with the idea that this might take time to work through. All these changes help to create better health and greater sustainability.

Sodium / Potassium and Acid / Alkaline Balances

These chemical balances in our foods and our bodies are two important practical guides to gaining true natural health. If you can get these balances right in a diet, whatever the proportions of cooked and raw foods, then you will be taking great strides to natural health and vitality.

These balances are highlighted in a great many raw food nutrition books, as well as many other natural health and healthy eating books, because they are key factors in maintaining the healthy activity and balance of the cells that make up our body – in our organs, in our blood, in our nervous system... in every part of our body in fact. So if you keep your cells healthy, you keep your body healthy.

Sodium and potassium work with each other when they are in a healthy balance – and when they are out of balance they work against each other. They are vital for maintaining a good state of health in cells, because they determine the osmotic pressure of the fluids both inside and outside the cells. And this is critical to health because it is the ability of the cells to pass unwanted and toxic materials out through these liquids that is vital in maintaining health. If the pressure is wrong then the cell cannot get these undesirables out, and they get stuck with them. Over time this leads to the degeneration of those cells.

Potassium has a number of important roles in the body, which are well detailed in The New Raw Energy, by Susannah and Leslie Kenton, and many other raw food nutrition books. Most western diets are high in inorganic sodium (i.e. table/rock salt or sea salt) and low in potassium, and for this reason our cells and bodies are unable to cleanse themselves in their natural, healthy way. However, if you want to keep things simple all you really need to know is what foods are good to eat to get your (organically bound) sodium and potassium balance right. As most western diets contain an excess of sodium (particularly because of being higher in 'table salt'), the main thing to do is to eat more potassium foods, and cut out table/rock salt and highly salted foods.

In his books *The Sunfood Diet Success System* and *Eating for Beauty*, David Wolfe provides much detail on the mineral contents of various foods. To get good levels of potassium you need to eat more green leafy vegetables, celery, most fruits especially apples, avocados, bananas, dates, durian, persimmon or kaki (with seeds), and pumpkin, as well as dried fruit; raisins with seeds, prunes and apricots. Macadamia nuts and sunflower seeds are also good potassium sources.

You also need to make sure your organic sources of sodium are healthy sources. This means green leafy vegetables, and particularly celery, kale and spinach, with seaweed being another good source. Fortunately celery, kale and spinach are all easy to grow in a wide range of climates (they all grow very well under our orange trees in southern Spain), so you can create your own organic sources of these minerals quite quickly. Chard leaf stems are also very high in sodium, and are great to use minced or chopped finely into patés and other dishes to get that salty flavour.

A word or five on inorganic table/rock salt... it is not a food! It is not a food because it provides no nutrition whatsoever. In fact, as Frederic Paténaude points out, it is actually toxic to the body: *"Salt kills life which is why we preserve foods in salt – it prevents living activity from occurring. It is an anti-biotic, which means 'anti-life'... It causes the body to retain water in order to dilute the salt in the tissues, and to prevent harming the cells."* Just so you know!

Salt is often a tough thing to give up, so allow yourself time by eating more of the naturally sodium rich foods, so that your salt-cravings go down. Use more seaweeds instead of salt, and make sure you do not over eat on the olives! Make sure they are organic and rinse them in unsalted water before eating them. Switch to high quality sea-salt if you continue using salt, and start by using less than half as much as you are used to, have many meals without any salt at all (i.e. fruit meals), or only add it in to a salad when you have eaten most of it already. The clear objective though should be to remove inorganic salt from your diet.

David Wolfe also cites the 12 year Schupan study of the nutritional superiority of organic vegetables, which found that organic produce has between 2 to 10 times higher mineral content than non-organic. This is a very powerful argument for growing your own organic produce – to maximise the mineral content, which is achieved by eating the produce as fresh as possible, straight from the garden.

With regard to the acid-alkaline balance, the natural state for the body and blood, to maintain natural, vibrant health, is slightly alkaline. The normal western diet is highly acid forming, with grains, meat and dairy produce being particular culprits. The body can survive if it is acid, but not in a truly healthy state. If your blood becomes acid you die very quickly. So the body struggles with the typical western diet, constantly maintaining the blood's alkalinity, but only by draining the body of its minerals, and maintaining acidity elsewhere in the body. This is the best it can do because it doesn't have the mineral rich, alkalising foods coming into the body. Dr Joel Robbins' tapes *Health Through Nutrition* explain the acid-alkaline balance particularly well.

Linked with the foods it takes in, the body often craves quick-hit alkalisers to balance its acidity – and it just so happens that the powerful alkaloids of coffee, tobacco and drugs have this effect. But after their immediate hit, their net effect is very much to maintain acidity, through the chain of reactions they cause in the body and appetite. But at least understanding that this is part of the cycle of cravings can help to break that cycle, because if you start to eat many highly alkalising foods your cravings for these addictive acid-causing alkaloids will fall off.

An acid body leads to degeneration of the cells, inside and out, because as every one knows acids eat away at things. We do need acids in our body, for example to help break down our food, however, the balance of alkaline to acid has to be around 80% alkaline to 20% acid if we are to maintain true vital health. Again, looking at our natural diet tells us what balance of foods will naturally, automatically create a good acid/alkaline balance. And that means organic raw fruits and vegetables... which will automatically give you the right sodium-potassium balance too. Raw foods that are acid forming and which therefore need to be eaten in moderation, and eaten with highly alkalising foods, are nuts and seeds, and avocados. Soaked nuts and seeds (soaked overnight, and then drained and rinsed) are less acid forming than if they are unsoaked.

So eat more alkaline foods, particularly green leafy vegetables, including wild greens, celery and cucumber. Other alkaline fruits if they are ripe (and remember most supermarket foods are not ripe) include figs, sun dried and unsalted black olives, grapefruit, lemon and citrus fruit in general, grapes with seeds, and papaya. Wild and organic fruit is definitely best, while overly sweet, hybridised fruits are basically more acid forming because of the unnaturally high levels of sugars.

The solution is easy in terms of knowing what to eat: more fresh, raw, organic fruits and vegetables, particularly making sure you have some green leafy vegetables, such as spinach and kale, or celery. What is not so easy is how to make these changes in what you eat, so that is what we need to look at next.

Taking Care of Yourself in the Short and Long Term: Maintaining Balance

The long term effects of more raw foods or a wholly raw food diet are variable, depending on each person's experiences and emotional patterns, both before and after 'getting into' raw food. Generally, however, it is unquestionable that the effects tend to be very much on the positive side.

The most widespread experience for high percentage raw foodists seems to be that of becoming more sensitive, often in all sorts of ways. Sensitivity to taste and smell, and other bodily reactions to food and environment are the most obvious areas. However, there are other areas that are very important to be aware of:

✳ Emotional sensitivity often rises, although this does not necessarily mean there is any greater emotional imbalance. What seems to happen is that one's 'senses' (from first to sixth and beyond!) generally become more 'sensitive'. So when feelings arise they are usually clearer and more direct. This can be seen as a clearer manifestation of 'emotional intelligence', provided one is not disconcerted by this sometimes sudden and possibly overwhelming increase in sensitivity. To me this is where emotions are a very important pointer from the mind-body to a situation of physical or emotional discomfort, or natural imbalance. So it is important to try to ensure that you have a lifestyle and/or circle of friends that can help you cope with that, in case it catches you by surprise!

✳ Sensitivity to air-borne pollution – this was very obvious to me when I first went raw when living in the city of Leicester (UK). When cycling to work each morning I found it increasingly difficult to tolerate the effects of the traffic pollution on my throat and on how I felt generally. My throat became mildly sore within a few minutes of cycling in traffic; this would gradually disappear over half-an-hour or so, once I had arrived at work.

✳ Sensitivity to noise and the urban lifestyle, particularly in the longer term. Generally many raw fooders find themselves less tolerant of the noise, bustle and harshness of large towns and cities, and feel more drawn to a more peaceful, natural lifestyle. However, like everyone else most raw fooders still live in towns and cities, so for many the health and energy benefits they feel can often give them more 'get up and go' even in an urban lifestyle.

✳ Intolerance to other diets and lifestyles. This can be a tough one, as going raw often make you think that everyone else's diet is almost insane; not even 'food'. This is the 'Why can't they see' syndrome and it is not an uncommon reaction to some of the revelations that often arise from going raw. The important point is that on the whole, what ever you believe it is normally NOT very effective if you go around trying to convert everyone, and being intolerant of other people's diets. If you want to demonstrate the benefits that you believe come from a raw food diet do it by example, not by preaching, arguing or intolerance to 'normal' diets.

By whatever route, when people discover the apparent seriousness of the world's social and ecological problems, including its health/sickness problems, aggression and anger can emerge, along with many other emotions. Discovering raw food nutrition or permaculture will certainly open your eyes to many things.

One of the side effects of a raw food lifestyle is certainly becoming more sensitive – in taste, tolerance to pollution and often in emotions, including sensitivity to joyous experiences, as well as sensing the less joyful aspects of human existence. This is partly through increased awareness of the range of lifestyle choices that are available. Anyone whose life experience has made them susceptible to aggression (which sadly is fairly common in our society) will probably feel more sensitive, and this sensitivity sometimes may be manifested as anger and even aggression.

Anger can be an appropriate and understandable response to the kinds of 'crimes against nature and humanity' that we see around the world; but if that anger becomes aggression it only worsens the problem. If anger emerges then you have to work to channel that anger positively, in ways that are not aggressive or violent, either physically or emotionally.

The other end of the extreme is also possible. Those who already have an abhorrence of violence and aggression will often become even more sensitive, which can result in increased difficulty living within a world that is often very violent, harsh and aggressive to one's senses. If you already feel alienated in the modern world then eating a lot more raw food is not going to lessen that feeling (unless you can find a community of raw fooders[48]). A raw food lifestyle may take you to a point where you feel desperate to change your living situation to one that feels more in harmony with your senses, your true nature, and to be with similar people. The sense of desperation will not be pleasant if you are isolated, but if you follow things through and make positive changes in your living situation that desperation can be replaced with something much more pleasant.

This is one of the points about combining the raw food and permaculture perspectives. Your whole lifestyle situation needs to be looked at, with diet as just a part of it. Where are you now and where are you heading? Where do you really want to be and what are the practical steps towards getting you there? It is usually best to ensure you are not physically and emotionally isolated if you are making any major lifestyle change.

So, on the whole, raw fooders' experiences suggest that a raw food diet is much more likely to reduce aggression than increase it. This is partly because of reduced acidity in the body linked with moving from a high protein diet – because acidity aggravates any feelings of stress and tension. This is particularly common in moving from a meat-eating diet, because such a change in diet is

---

[48] See appendix 2 on page 151 if you are interested in raw eco-communities like Ecoforest.

known to effect bodily acidity and hormone balances. It is also because of the raw foods containing key nutrients and trace elements that are lacking in a 'normal' diet. This is demonstrated by the research of The Behavioural Health Partnership, which studied aggressive and other dysfunctional behaviour in military trainees and criminals, and found that significant improvement in diet lead to significant improvements in behaviour[49]. Many vegans have also found that they tend to feel less aggressive about animal rights issues, whilst feeling equally strongly – they see that violent attitudes towards human animals are no better than violent attitudes towards other animals.

Whether the subject is diet or permaculture, or both, if you are trying to provide more information to people so that they have more options in making their lifestyle choices, it does not normally work if you make someone feel wrong or go around attacking their diet or lifestyle. Whether you are talking about diet or organics, more times than not, such an approach will lead to an understandably defensive response to your attack. It is better just to be yourself and be as comfortable as you can living your own life in what ever way feels right to you. The more at ease you are with your diet the more people will be open, interested and inquiring about what you eat and your general lifestyle.

Intolerance of other perspectives is fairly common in anyone who thinks or feels that they have found 'THE' answer. And it is not uncommon for raw foodies to think raw food is 'THE' answer. Beware of this because it will normally lead to feeling very frustrated when others 'just don't get it'. I have seen this in permaculture people, vegans and raw foodies that feel they have 'seen the light'. I would never suggest that raw food or permaculture is the one answer to all the world's problems, and I do not tend to feel comfortable with those that do. Raw food fundamentalism or permaculture fundamentalism may be more positive, less unhealthy and more sustainable – but it is not balanced. To me the most impressive advocates of any movement or philosophy are those that express compassion, tolerance and understanding, with an inner self-confidence and certainty. Such people never preach, they just do.

What I see and feel is that diet and lifestyle, including what food we grow, is part of a huge web of inter-connected effects. Changing your diet and lifestyle will have very significant effects. This includes reactions to other people, what they say and how they behave, as well as reactions to your own lifestyle and the world around you. Finding a more positive diet and lifestyle is important but do not expect fundamental changes to be an instant answer to all your problems, or all the problems of the world.

Loren Lockman suggests that there are different levels of health:

✳ Transitional health: with many positive effects including higher energy, noticeable differences, feeling much better, etc., and with differing degrees of cleansing and detoxification still required for optimum levels of health.

---

[49] See www.restorative-health.co.uk and the booklet *Writings on Nutrition and Behaviour*, BHP, Outalong, Lower Broad Oak Road, West Hill, Ottery St Mary, Devon EX11 1XH, UK.

* Vibrant health: it will normally take some time to achieve truly vibrant health. Transitional health will feel very good in comparison with 'normal' health, and is the necessary step towards vibrant health.

Assimilation is the key thing... over-eating inhibits assimilation; too much fat and protein inhibits assimilation; stress inhibits assimilation. Being relaxed, eating when you are hungry, rather than to satisfy appetite and cravings, and having a good balance of primarily fruits and vegetables, with perhaps some nuts and seeds in good combinations, will ensure that you are on the path towards much improved assimilation.

Whatever route you take you will experience change, and that can be fascinating in itself. These days many mystics and scientists say the same thing about the nature of nature; that chaos reigns (although this is not 'chaos' in a negative sense). Getting a feel for nature and chaos will give you a stronger sense of how positive changes in your own lifestyle will effect positive and often subtle changes in the wider whole. The true meaning of chaos is an ever moving complexity of inter-related effects, which includes a fundamental degree of uncertainty. So any major evolution – or revolution – in your lifestyle, or in a whole society, will throw out a whole range of unexpected effects. So if you do make rapid changes in your life, do 'expect the unexpected', as they say.

Raw Parenting

Information sources and books to help parents and children with more naturally healthy and enjoyable lifestyles are growing in number all the time – these are designed to help those that are wanting to eat a lot more raw foods and 'transitioning', as well those that wish to create a 100% raw family lifestyle. Some of the excellent resources that are now available are listed in the resources section of this book.

There are a whole number of issues that parents meet when transitioning a family to more raw foods. As I am not a parent I am not an expert in this area although I have observed and know a few that are – so I know it is nothing to fear and it is a positive path to follow. There are several things that can help:

* The state of mind of the parent is by far the most important thing: younger kids copy parents, teenagers need freedom. If you are at ease with the changes and with your lifestyle, excited by them, enthusiastic about them and so on, then the children, particularly younger children will be too. Focus on your own mental attitude and emotions if you want the kids to enjoy a more natural and healthy way of living. Be creative, make it a game and an adventure, and also make sure it is something that gives them (and you) a sense of security, confidence and love.

* Colourful and interesting looking foods, as well as delicious foods, obviously help a lot. There is a fantastic range of recipes now available that are ideally suited to children – again see the resources section.

But don't worry about kids not enjoying the food or finding it boring – there are many now who have gone through this process, and a great number of parents find that their children really love raw and living foods. The earlier they start the better of course, and there can be challenges if kids have already got into junk foods. You can be confident that there is a great deal of good experience, guidance and support now there for you, and that it usually turns out to be a wonderful and positive experience for both children and parents alike.

* Children detox much more directly, and in a more matter of fact way. Most kids on a 'normal' diet get horrible colds and mucus anyway. The detox process will clear this out, which will not feel any different to a bad cold to the child, and leaving them much clearer, with little or no mucus depending on the degree and type of raw foods they eat, and what else they eat. If they eat 50% raw and 50% junk they will be very 'snotty'; if they eat 50% raw or more, and the rest is carefully selected cooked wholefoods they will be in good shape, provided they eat little or no dairy or wheat – the two big mucus producers. There are challenges for single parents when the other parent is not supportive of the raw diet. In these situations it is much better to be clear that you just want the child to eat more healthily, with a lot of fruit and raw vegetables, and to cut out junk foods. It may make things more difficult if you talk about going all raw.

* Inventing your own recipes with the kids is great fun for all involved, and is much easier than cooked recipes. Also you can be confident with raw sweets, and be happy knowing they are really healthy for your children, giving them the high quality nutrition they need – rather than 'normal' sweets, snacks, cakes and biscuits which can be really damaging to their teeth, create hyperactivity or be potentially fattening and addictive.

* With salads, get the kids involved in growing the salads – and making them. They will learn and be excited by this in itself, they will also make the direct connection with the food, and will be much more excited about eating salads when they have grown or helped to grow them themselves.

* Generally, you can use the whole process of change as an education process, helping the kids to understand where their food comes from geographically and from what types of plants, how it is grown, and how it makes the body naturally healthy.

The books on raw parenting that are listed in the appendices give a great deal of advice based on genuine personal experiences. They also give a wide range of excellent recipes designed to excite the taste and meet the nutritional needs of children. Rather than attempting to address all the issues here, I recommend that parents do some research themselves and take advantage of the books and contacts listed in the appendices so that they can learn from experienced experts.

To Create Healthy People and a Healthy Planet

Avoid Wheat and Grains: Why?

✳ Grains are just not a natural food for human beings and are not good for you as a food.

✳ Wheat is addictive and grains are acidifying for the body, creating lots of mucus, and adding to the mucoid plaque in your colon (particularly when combined with fats), which then inhibits the assimilation of nutrition of other foods into your body.

✳ Wheat growing is turning unimaginably vast areas of the world into desert, killing the soil.

✳ To grow it creates vast mono-cultures and is anti-ecology, anti-nature.

✳ It is creating a horrendous economic, chemical and psychological dependency amongst the farmers that grow it.

Avoid Milk and Meat: Why?

✳ Commercially/industrially farmed animals generally have vast amounts of drugs, vaccinations, and so on pumped into them (because they are so unhealthy being farmed in this way), which becomes concentrated in their flesh and in their milk. Eating animal flesh or milk products, cheese, yoghurt, etc means you are taking these drugs, vaccinations and so on into your body in a concentrated form.

✳ In Britain, and similarly in other western nations, 80% to 90% of arable land is used to grow crops for animal fodder, when we would need a lot less arable land if we were just growing plant foods for humans to eat, thus releasing a great deal of land for nature, reducing the demand for and therefore the cost of land.

✳ Generally flesh and milk products are acid and mucus forming in the body.

Avoid Vaccinations: Why?

✳ The threat of the diseases that we are told vaccinations protect us from may not always be as great as we are led to believe.

✳ In some cases the dangers of serious side effects from the vaccinations may be higher than the danger from the diseases themselves.

✳ Vaccinations are normally made with animal products in them.

✳ Vaccinations are unnatural materials in our bodies and create significant emotional and mental disturbances as a result.

Some Frequently Asked Questions About Eating More Raw Foods

This is all very inspiring, but I don't want to go 100% raw.

How do I go to 50:50, 50% raw, 50% cooked? How is this best achieved? What foods should I eat and when?

The very first thing to do to get to 50% raw is to just have fresh fruit for breakfast and if you feel hungry snack on fruit during the morning. For really active people Dr Douglas Graham recommends really filling up on fruit – and he means just fruit – for breakfast. Again it's a matter of trying a few things, but generally you can be confident that fruit only mornings is the best first step and will give you a real feeling of heightened energy and clarity early on.

In addition to the fruit only mornings ideally you need to: a) have one type of ripe fresh fruit at least 30 minutes before other meals (because ripe fruit digests quickly), and/or b) with non-fruit meals, as much as possible have a salad of raw vegetables as the first part of every main meal, and at least a salad of raw vegetables as part of every main meal. These should not be boring old lettuce, cucumber, tomato and onion salads unless you particularly like that! If you have a raw lunch too you will also notice quite quickly that that well-known after lunch drowsiness that hits so many people at work just is not there any more.

As mentioned elsewhere in the book, first get off fried foods, junk foods and processed foods completely. It really is not at all difficult to get to 50% raw or more, you just need to take a look at some of the raw recipes in this book and others, and see what takes your fancy. Also simply understand that if you get comfortable and confident with about 10 or 15 different basic salad ingredients – some being particular favourites of yours – then you can constantly change the mixes, proportions and combinations of these, with a few other exotic ingredients when you feel like it and (surprisingly perhaps) then you'll find that every salad tastes different. And I'll bet that you'll find that you're less bored than with your previous diet! Ideally, make sure at least two meals a day are completely raw.

Will the food be satisfying enough?

The simple answer is 'yes'... when you learn what satisfies you. The initial transition to eating more raw foods is when you may worry most about being satisfied. Sprouted chick pea humous, seed or nut dips and seed patés are all satisfying foods. Dried fruit, nuts and seeds, and the more fatty foods are good fillers too. After trying many things one family that visited us at Ecoforest – Zohar and Nitzana and their four boys – have found that eating fruit before a main salad meal leads to satisfaction for them.

A carpenter who works long days in London and who visited us at Ecoforest having been vegan for 20 years before, has found that a very large fruit salad with plenty of bananas and some tahini mixed in, really keeps him satisfied right through the day, until he gets back home for an evening salad.

Many people find (our carpenter friend Alex included) that fairly soon after switching to eating all or mainly raw they actually are not wanting to eat so much. This is a natural change because the food they are eating actually has a lot more nutrition in it – so they can get the same nutrition whilst needing to eat less, which means they feel more satisfied, not less satisfied eating raw foods. This is also particularly noticeable if you switch to eating all or mainly organic foods... as well as if you remember to chew your food properly too.

Three relatively harmless bulk cooked foods are potatoes (steamed), oats and millet. These foods require relatively little processing, and energy to cook. Organic rolled oats (normally heat dried, therefore not raw) are acidifying but can be used in moderation if soaked in water and uncooked. Millet requires very little processing and can be cooked just by bringing to the boil and then turning the heat off and leaving it for 5 to 10 minutes. It is also a relatively healthy cooked food as it is the only alkaline grain. These were foods that I ate as basic fillers when I was transitioning to raw foods. Basically, if you substitute these and other foods for bread, meat and dairy, even if you don't eat much more raw food you will be doing yourself and the planet a great deal of good. Along with steamed vegetables they are relatively harmless cooked food fillers.

Remember not to combine badly, particularly if you are still eating cooked starches.

What is a typical diet for a week? And what do I do about sourcing all the ingredients...?

A typical diet for a week? Again a good and understandable question but then we need to know whose typical diet you mean? We also need to know what time of the year? For example, do most people eat the same in the depths of winter as they do in the summer? What climate are they in? Do they grow some of their own food? Do they buy from an organic veggie box scheme, a local market or do they buy mail-order or from a supermarket?

Self-confidence and confidence in your foods and your own creative ability is my recipe for health. Whilst it's a good question, there is of course no such thing as a typical person or a typical week – so I don't want to give you a menu plan that might not suit your tastes and needs. I want you to know that you can explore and experiment and find out what suits you – and you will learn and have fun in the process. But I also have some helpful hints.

To start with buy more of a variety of fruit and veg than you might normally do – and then pick what you fancy for breakfast, lunch and at supper time, perhaps with intent of trying a raw humous, or seed paté for supper, or some avocado dish with whatever salad you choose to create for lunch, and a decent fruit breakfast (Dr Douglas Graham recommends bananas in particular). Make sure your week's food supply includes a number of options for raw fats, sugars and proteins but remember that *greens* are the best source for building proteins and you don't need lots and lots of nuts and seeds, or other concentrated proteins.

Most people do well with fruit for breakfast and as morning snacks, with some preferring fruit lunches too with a salad in the evening. Others prefer main salads for lunch and fruit in the evening, and some a salad for both lunch and supper. I started with fruit in the morning and salads for lunch and supper, and then at about 4 to 6 months I naturally shifted to a fruit lunch too, with a salad just in the evening. This has been my basic pattern for over eight years now, with a few variations here and there, depending on how I feel at the time. And I always know that whatever balance I feel like, it's good for me.

As far as sourcing goes, one approach (if you can afford it) is to buy virtually everything from Nature's First Law (USA) or from the Fresh Network, Orkos and/or Organics Direct (UK/Europe) by mail order... It is good for many people that this option is available, but it is not necessarily a recommendation because it's hardly local sourcing, and is high on 'food miles'! I suggest that your local organic veggie box scheme, organic farm shops and wholefood stores are your greatest resources, along with your garden, backyard, or allotment, and then there's farmer's markets and regular markets too – and local wholesalers, who often have ripe fruit at really good prices. You have the choice to go for what suits you – if you like over the phone, mail order and bulk buying then there are the organisations out there that will provide very high quality food and make it very easy for you. And if you prefer it fresh and local, there's normally people out there to do that too. And if you like a bit of both then go for that.

What I really do *not* recommend is your local supermarket. Supermarkets sell what suits them, not what suits you. Very often it's not ripe or good quality in terms of its nutritional value even if it looks spotless and shiny. Supermarkets tend to destroy local food markets and supply networks. They encourage you to drive, and the vast, vast majority of the stuff they sell as 'food' (i.e. row after row of processed and package 'garbage' food) is actively creating or sustaining illness and disease more than health. So if you buy from supermarkets you are supporting the profits of those that sell foods that tend to create illness and disease rather than health. That's that little rant done with!

How do you stop a raw diet/lifestyle becoming boring?
Well, that's a good and interesting question isn't it? And my immediate answer is; well, how do you stop a cooked food diet/lifestyle becoming boring?! It's easy – you make your food interesting and enjoyable, which is easy with raw foods. There's a vast array of different foods, recipes, combinations, super simple approaches or complex 'cordon bleu' approaches and so on that you can try. Raw foods are definitely no more boring than cooked foods and have at least as many opportunities for creativity and awesome, amazing flavour experiences. In fact, generally it seems that people find that once they are eating a lot of raw foods they can taste 'a lot more and a lot better', and therefore they enjoy their food more. This is because the taste system becomes cleansed and because the taste of raw foods is really fresh and alive. Also it's easier to experiment with raw foods, as it's difficult to make raw disasters – whereas

cooked disasters are much easier to achieve!

To avoid boredom it's basically up to you, and it's easy to avoid boredom. There are plenty of subtle or spicy flavours to play with, and a whole host of exciting food combinations to explore. On the fruit side you can try deliciously simple mixes like orange or grapefruit and avocado, apple and avocado, or banana and avocado – or you can go for much more complex dishes. Then on the salad or main meal side try a raw curry, carrot and ginger, grated carrot and orange, or believe it or not, finely chopped leek and grated parsnip with a little olive oil and a dash of tamari is delicious. Using different seaweeds in salads, raw vegan 'sushi'/nori rolls and other dishes provides yet another dimension to taste experiments.

Personally I'm not really into recipes – I like to just create what I feel like at the time, and I get great results like this. However, to make life simpler for you, the eager reader, there are a number of recipes included in the appendices section of this book to help you out if you do want to try some. They are chosen to be relatively simple, and many have been donated by people who have been through the transition experience themselves, and their offerings are carefully selected to aid that process – both in terms of the nutrition they offer and the variety of flavours and textures, as well as the look of the food – which is also often much more appealing when you get the hang of raw foods than that same old rather dreary cycle of standard cooked dishes.

What extra equipment would I need? Is a juicer essential?
The only things that are essential are a knife, a bowl and a chopping board... and even they are optional for some! Having a juicer can be an excellent investment, but is not essential. Juicing speeds up the cleansing process. Food processors are used by many people – but remember that hand processors, such as a hand mincer or seed grinder, or even a pestle and mortar, are often at least as good as electric, and far more ecological. Hand mincers and seed grinders are great for seed patés, raw cakes and raw curries – a whole host of dishes in fact. And these hand powered devices are readily available from the FRESH Network, Nature's First Law and Living Nutrition.

But, you don't actually need any of these things. Some of the greatest, most amazing salads and other dishes are easily produced by hand. Don't switch from a cooker dependency to a blender dependency – simplicity is safe, enjoyable and delicious! The simplest implements are... quite simply the simplest implements.

What are the best things to sprout?
In my experience some of the best and simplest things to sprout are green lentils and chickpeas, with sunflower seeds being excellent if you have a good quality supply (if they are not good quality they will rot quite quickly once soaked). Quinoa, aduki beans and alfalfa are also excellent, and you will find that different sprouts have different characters and that you will use them

in different ways in a meal. For example, you will find that alfalfa and quinoa are great mixed in with greens, or other salad elements, with chickpeas being great to use in humous as a satisfying, staple part of the salad. I tend to find mung beans (which are the bean sprouts most often available in shops) to be troublesome, as not all sprout and some stay very hard, creating a bit of a surprise and quite a crunch for the teeth. Lentils of different sorts all tend to be simple, and taste excellent. Radish, mustard and fenugreek are great if you want something with a bit more zap to it!

Sprouts are an excellent way to get really high quality organic nutrition at a very, very low cost, and I recommend this for individuals and families on a low budget, as well as for students. It can be great fun getting a sprouting system going, and whilst it might seem a little daunting at first, like most of the raw lifestyle, it is actually very easy and enjoyable once you get going. But be aware that sprouts are *not* an essential raw food. With a well designed diet we can definitely get all our nutritional needs without them. The Ann Wigmore school of raw foodists do promote them. Meanwhile the hygienists do not see them as a natural food for us – except in limited quantities of sprouted greens (e.g. just the green shoots of sprouted sunflower seeds, which are delicious), as opposed to eating the whole range of sprouted pulses, beans, etc.

The basics of sprouting are: most things need to soak overnight, no longer, then drained, and then rinsed once or twice a day – they will normally be ready between 2 and 4 days. There are some excellent and cheap books on sprouting available from the main raw/living foods networks, such as Edward Kearney's *The Sprouting Handbook* (see page 154 for network details).

What do you eat when you visit friends and family?

Personally, when I visit friends and family, or go out to a restaurant I have a very simple and effective strategy – I just tell people what I want.

I am always totally willing to bring my own food, and often I even prepare meals for my friends with them, in their houses (which I enjoy doing and which they seem to enjoy too) as they are usually keen to try something new, interesting and different. Obviously this depends on what your friends are like, and I may be lucky to have particularly open and interested friends. Just making clear what I do eat (rather than what I do not eat) often makes it really simple, and it seems that a raw vegetable salad is quite easily understandable by most people – more so than requesting a cooked vegan or macrobiotic meal for example.

When visiting my family (parents) they are accepting of my choices. Whilst at first I found it difficult at times to eat alongside their meat or fish and cooked veg meals (mainly because of my own unnecessary defensiveness about what I was doing), it has also been a question of me adapting to them as well as them adapting to my changes. They now usually enjoy sharing some of my exotic salad concoctions as part of their meals, and are always happy to buy in a few extra salad ingredients if they know I am coming to visit. Again, maybe I am lucky with my parents, and not all may be so understanding. The main thing is to be content with what you are doing in yourself, and to be clear that you enjoy it and feel better for it. Like lots of things, it may be useful to give it time to evolve in its own way. Most parents want to see their children healthy and happy, so whilst some parents will definitely worry about what you are doing, in time they will see that you are healthier and happier.

When it comes to partners and/or children this can be a more complex issue that I have not had to deal with along my path (my partners since becoming raw have all been either 100% or a high percentage raw). This can be a sticky and challenging issue for some, whilst for others it brings closer understanding and connection. Again, the main thing is to be clear in yourself and to be doing what feels right to you, within the context of the relationship. Some of the raw food networks, books and magazines can be useful in providing advice if you feel in need of more information or some support.

When visiting restaurants and/or pubs for meals I have found that in virtually all cases they seem to enjoy the opportunity to prepare something different, although I always emphasise 'just vegetables and fruit, all raw is what I want – nothing cooked, and with no salad dressings, egg or cheese thank you'. Asking for a simple avocado salad seems to be the best strategy. Although some do not rise to the challenge, in general I have enjoyed some fantastic salads with this simple, clear request. I often carry a couple of apples with me if I go out, just in case I get the somewhat sad lettuce, cucumber, tomato and onion cliché salad!

What are the best things to drink and how important are they?
In some ways your foods become your drinks, especially where fruits are concerned. In terms of liquids though, water is best and ideally spring water fresh from a spring – then bottled spring water (still, not gassed) is next best. Fresh juices (vegetable and fruit juices) are also excellent – and by 'fresh' I mean only freshly made by you or your host, and I do not mean bought juices that are labelled as 'fresh'. (If you have to drink tap water then it should be left to stand for some time to allow the chlorine to evaporate off.)

It is important to have plenty of liquid in your diet, but that does not necessarily mean drinking a lot. Remember you're eating foods with a lot more liquids in them when you eat more raw foods. If you are not 100% raw (and only a small proportion are) inevitably that also means you're eating some cooked foods. These are normally dehydrating, and therefore cause you to want to drink – like salty foods, breads and biscuits and so on. If possible satisfy your thirst with water, fresh juice or fruit, although you need to avoid bad combinations if you go for the juicy fruit option. I have found that apples are good thirst quenchers that can be eaten comfortably at all times and after most other foods if I am thirsty.

Some people seem to drink more than others and I'm in that category – I think this often is more of a habit than a biological necessity. Spring water with a little freshly squeezed lemon or orange juice is my favourite. If you want a hot drink herb teas are best (ideally fresh herbs of course), or plain hot water. Personally I rarely drink these now and tend to feel better without them, because the very high temperature of the drink feels very unnatural to me, and definitely does the mouth, throat and digestive system no good.

As far as other standard drinks in our society go let's start with coffee... because I know a lot about it! And because it's a tough bean to crack! Coffee is a very hard and harsh drug to the system, that will very probably lead to severe de-mineralisation of your body if it is drunk in significant quantities over time (e.g. 2 or more cups per day for a number of years). If you are all or mainly raw the effects of coffee are more severe... This I know from my own harsh experience of having been something of a caffeine-head. If you want to give up coffee, using organic cocoa is a good transition with much lower caffeine levels. Often sugar addiction is part and parcel of the coffee addiction, so if you are struggling to give such things up be aware that it can be a tough one (for many but not all), so be compassionate with yourself. Feel some understanding for your addictions!

Tea is not really any better than coffee, although shifting to weak black tea can be a pleasant change, whereas shifting to weak black coffee ain't so satisfying! Tea also contains significant caffeine, as well as tannin which inhibits digestion. Again, like coffee, if you are used to drinking a lot of tea either give it up completely if you can, or give yourself time and allow a gradual transition if you need to – perhaps use the weak black tea option if you need to.

In my humble opinion, drinks like Coca Cola, Pepsi and other canned and bottled sweet and fizzy drinks are quite simply appalling for your health from a natural, living/raw food perspective, (as well as being environmentally appalling) and they should be assigned to the past as soon as possible. I have nothing more to say on these junk drinks, except that even those that masquerade as being healthy are not.

Alcohol is for you to deal with as you see fit. It has a huge social role in western society, although it is also one of the biggest killers and creators of illness and addiction, personal and family problems and unhappiness. More and more people are living without, or with very little alcohol, and having a great time without it. Certainly your relationship with alcohol, if you have one, is likely to change as you eat more raw foods. Red wine in smaller quantities is probably most acceptable from the raw perspective, ideally organic if bought, and even better would be home-made or locally made fruit wines from berries or other fruit such as plums. Local real ale or cider would be the best option if you really love your beer, or want to carry on with it in social situations. From an environmental standpoint I always point out that any alcohol made from fruit is far, far better than one made from grain.

Let's Be Honest – Are there any dangers?

Well to answer this one, I want to emphasise that very few ask this question from a 'level playing field', which means they tend to forget the very real dangers of a normal western diet. Look at the statistics and trends for health that reflect the effects of a 'normal' diet first. As with any diet or lifestyle, there are a few dangers with the raw lifestyle, a few of these are physical, and some are emotional/psychological... but they are fewer and far less dangerous than sticking with the standard western diet.

B12 Deficiency

B12 deficiency is something that is important to be aware of – and my views on this have evolved over time through my own experience and through observing other vegan raw food eaters over time. As far as I know most of those I know that eat a lot of raw foods do not have and have not had any B12 problems – although some I know have. We are not living a 'natural' life, eating in 'natural' ways, therefore we are not gaining our 'natural' sources of B12, which are bacteria on plants and fruit, and the occasional insect grub in fruit in particular.

One of the most important aspects with B12 is assimilation – in other words what B12 (and other nutrients) your body is able to take in through the digestive system, rather than the amount of B12 you consume. This is an issue for your nutrition in general and for trace elements in particular, and it depends on the amount of undesirable material you have shifted from your system (i.e. mucoid plaque) – and this normally requires some fasting, juice fasting, herbal cleanses or colonics.

We have to have B12 for proper brain function, and to me it is much better to take the occasional B12 tablet or from time to time or use some yeast extract in some otherwise raw dishes to avoid the risk of B12 deficiency... because B12 deficiency is not fun. You lose your sense of direction and feel 'all over the place' with B12 deficiency – lost, disempowered and unable to focus or concentrate. So be aware of the potential for B12 deficiency and do something to avoid it if you want to. There is plenty of information about the B12 issue within the raw food networks, so you can always look into the issue more to help you make your own choice. You don't need to be afraid of it – but you do need to be aware of it and make sure you eat to avoid it.

Teeth...

Unless you are eating in a very natural way, with virtually all organic and wild foods, I would definitely recommend that you ignore any raw fooders or others that suggest you don't need to brush your teeth. We are all starting with non-ideal teeth, and from a lifetime of eating foods that are not good for the teeth, so most of our teeth and gums are not in great shape. Carry on looking after you teeth, and carry on brushing them – not after every meal or even twice a day necessarily, but definitely daily or regularly.

Be very careful about eating unripe fruit, and particularly lots of unripe oranges (fresh and ripe from the tree is a different story!). Supermarket oranges and much of the fruit that is sold in shops and supermarkets is sold for profit not for health. It is easier to transport and store, has fewer losses and lasts longer on the shelves for the supermarkets if it is not ripe... and if it isn't ripe it's definitely not good for the teeth, because it is more acid than nature intended it to be and the acid will attack the teeth and gums. Eating plenty of fresh, organic home grown greens (especially perennials, wild foods, etc.) is good for the health of your teeth and gums.

Frederic Paténaude, the editor of *Just Eat An Apple* magazine and author of *Raw Secrets* has written some excellent articles and a chapter in his book on the dangers of eating too many nuts[50]. Eating a lot of nuts creates too much acidity in the body and the mouth. This then robs the body of minerals in order to maintain the body's essential Ph balance. After much research on this issue Fred is certain that eating too many nuts and seeds (especially if not soaked or sprouted) is a major cause of the teeth problems that some raw fooders have experienced. He recommends no more than 100 grams per day. Dried fruits are concentrated sugars, as with any other concentrated sugar, excessive dried fruit can lead to teeth problems.

Apart from unripe fruit and too many nuts, most ripe and raw foods are either neutral or good for the teeth and gums. As with most things, balance is the key. And remember that all the starches and sugars of a so called 'normal' diet are at least as much of a danger as the raw alternatives.

Steve's Position on Raw Food
So what exactly is my position on the best balance of raw foods? Well, I don't have an exact position as such. But, I certainly feel and know from experience that eating a high proportion of fruit is what makes me feel best, with a regular dose of vibrant green vegetables. I feel that a high intake of fatty foods (avocados and oils, etc.) or high protein foods (nuts and seeds) does not make me feel so good. Salty foods (like salted olives) also definitely do not make me feel my best.

I also know that I feel at my best eating simply... whole natural fruit, just one type, straight from the tree is 'it'. I definitely feel my best eating one fruit at a time when I eat during the day, with a salad in the late afternoon or evening, or eating only fruit for several days at a time. Personally, I also feel excellent when I eat less, particularly when I just have water until say between 1pm and 3pm in the afternoon. This appears to work well even if I am doing physical work, although I tend to do this only when the weather is warm or hot where I live most of the time in Spain. I do believe that eating more than we need to is one of the main things that has greatly slowed or even blocked progress towards vibrant health for many on the raw path, myself included at times.

In general, I feel that we really know ourselves what is good for us if we listen to our body, and are honest with ourselves. If you want to follow a school of thought on your path to eating more raw foods then the hygienist perspective appears the most balanced to me as well as learning to 'listen' to your body. Allowing yourself time to transition may be important. Being clear and

[50] In both *JEAA* and *Get Fresh!* magazines, various 2002 editions.

motivated about your objective is also important. Listen to your body, listen to your emotions, listen to your mind and listen to your spirit – think about which of these are the best guide at different times. And really get into feeling the affects of your foods as you eat and digest them, and feel the changes as your body cleanses.

Psychological Stuff

Raw food is NOT, repeat NOT, the answer to life the universe and everything... It will normally make you feel more alive, more healthy and more energised. But it's not a panacea that will sort out the psychological and emotional problems, which actually seem to be at least as widespread in our society as the physical health problems that are often so much more directly visible, and certainly much more openly accepted and talked about.

Over-eating and bad food combinations can be common when emotional issues arise, or when toxins come into the system leading to cravings to eat things that will stop the detox process. Limiting your fats and protein (i.e. nuts and seeds) intake is important. Eating small amounts at such times will see you through, but you may need to control a desire to over-eat, which is generally the result of the culture habit of eating far more than we need. As Frederic Paténaude's book *Raw Secrets* emphasises more than any other recent raw food book, this is a desire to satisfy the appetite... which has nothing to do with real hunger. You will get a lot of comforting advice in some raw food books, but I recommend Fred's as one of the most clear, direct and honest on a whole range of these issues.

Some people can feel more isolated from normal society if they go raw, and sensitivity can increase in different ways. As well as detoxing physically there is normally some detoxing of emotional stuff that goes on. So much depends on your character and personality, your awareness of these issues, your self awareness and your personal strength in tackling any ups and downs that come up in the process, and the support around you (or lack of it).

Anyone needing psychiatric care or mental health support will probably get some benefits from eating more raw foods, particularly as research by the Behavioural Health Partnership and others suggests that many behavioural problems are directly linked to the typically poor western diet, that lacks essential vitamins and minerals which are needed for proper brain function. Going raw is not going to 'sort out' those psychological or emotional problems, although it will often help remove some of the key chemical causes that accentuate many psychological imbalances, and with children it will often help significantly.

There are many influences and effects on our psychology and emotions of course, and many psychological and emotional problems go right back to childhood. Eating more raw foods can lift off some of the layers that 'dumb down' some of our patterns, and at the same time it can help us to see and experience things more clearly, so that we understand ourselves better and give ourselves more choices about how to respond to or change those patterns.

It is for you to decide whether the above issues are real 'dangers' or perhaps more accurately merely issues to be aware of and then to take simple, sensible steps to avoid. Like a pot hole when you're cycling, it can be dangerous if you are cycling in the dark, but if you have the light of awareness shining ahead of you it is merely a hole in the path to avoid. The reality is that the real dangers lie in cancers and degenerative diseases, or rather in the causes of these degenerative diseases – the standard western lifestyle and diet. It is the causes of these degenerative diseases that you should be doing your utmost to avoid. Cancer cells are effectively mutated cells, and unlike normal cells which 'breathe' oxygen, cancer cells, like plants, 'breathe' carbon dioxide. Cooked food and a lack of circulation in the body's systems creates a carbon dioxide rich environment in the body that is ideal for the growth of cancer cells. Raw food is oxygen rich. Well balanced raw food nutrition, combined with other health creating activities as discussed in the next section, will ensure that you create an oxygen rich system, that welcomes in health, and pushes away the dangers of degenerative disease.

If you are at all worried about going completely raw I suggest you change to about 70-80% raw, and have 6 or more completely raw weeks each year, with perhaps 3-6 fasts of 3 days each year. This will certainly be a very positive change... if you give up wheat, meat and dairy that is, and other habits that are destructive for your health. Cutting right back on these at first is an option, although sometimes this can be used as an excuse for 'backsliding' or 'slippage'! But cutting right back is not avoiding the pot holes, it is just making the pot holes smaller.

You will find that the hygienist approach is probably the clearest and most helpful if you adopt this 70% or more raw approach. Be honest with yourself. Don't pretend you are going all raw if you are not – decide on how raw you really want to be and do it. And then whether you are going completely raw or not, make sure you are not over-eating, and make sure you have a well balanced diet. 70% raw fruits and vegetables, eating mainly steamed or lightly boiled starchy vegetables as your cooked foods, with no grains, meat or dairy, and eating sensible and not excessive quantities of nuts and dried fruit (or not eating them at all), will give you fantastic results.

I also recommend that you consider some of the other dimensions beyond diet and food that can contribute to creating more complete, whole health for yourself and others...

Meditation

Meditating is a perfect complement to a more ecological lifestyle. I suggest it would be a very important part of a 'lifestyle guild' for you, that includes growing your own organic food and eating a high proportion of raw plant foods. Meditation can be part of your daily diet that will help bring a more complete and more naturally clear and energized level of physical, mental, emotional and spiritual health.

From my own experience I know that meditation can have an incredibly powerful and positive effect on a person's life. I believe that you really need to learn to meditate from a good teacher – and make sure you have regular support, encouragement and advice for at least the first two months after learning. Without this you can learn the technique well, but then be left with unanswered questions and queries as the meditation starts to take effect over the first weeks and months, and as your perception and experience of life changes.

The most difficult thing about meditation is not the learning of the technique (that's normally fairly simple). Like the raw food transition, it's the changing of old patterns to new patterns that can be more difficult. Establishing a new timetable in your daily life is sometimes easy, and sometimes hard. Personally I started meditating when I moved to a new house and a new town, so it fitted in really well with starting some completely new patterns in my life. This can work well; to start meditating when there's another significant change happening in your life.

From my own experience I can recommend TM (Transcendental Meditation) as a technique, although it may not be right for everyone. It can be incredibly powerful and effective – and I mean 'incredible' in the literal sense, which is that it is not credible to the logical mind; the logical mind cannot accurately understand or imagine the effects. TM took me to a state of being in my everyday life that was just so positive, stress-free and creative. It really helped me to open up and see that I was not who I thought I was; so it really helped me change myself in a very positive way.

Some people do adopt a semi-religious approach to TM and other schools of meditation. Many people seem to feel more comfortable when strongly attached to or identifying with a single philosophy, personality or teacher. Whether it be politics, religion, a sport, or TM, permaculture or the raw food movement, there are always people that like to identify themselves with one dominant idea. This is more a reflection of people than anything to worry about with TM, permaculture or raw food. I feel that we all have equally huge potential, and the really frightening challenge is to face up to being your own guru, learning from a range of sources. Make your own choices about your relationship with TM, or any other form of meditation, philosophy or lifestyle choice. I feel that meditation, supported by teachers and meditation networks, can be a very positively and supremely healthy part of your life. And if you want to get more involved with TM or other schools of meditation you can. There are many fascinating courses run by the TM movement, such as Vedic Maths (which is a real eye opener for mathematicians and mathematical incompetents alike!). Meditation weekends and Vedic Science courses are also a great experience. It's also worth noting that the TM movement has been responsible for a vast amount of respected scientific research into the effects of meditation.

One of the great things about TM is it only takes 40 to 50 minutes a day (about 20 minutes each in the morning and in the evening). I slept much better and did things much more effectively, so I gained far, far more than those 40 to 50 minutes spent meditating. The now world famous Dr Deepak Chopra emerged from the TM movement and his early works are good sources of information about the beneficial effects of TM and the practice.

My own experiences with meditation included internal travels to places of freedom, openness and a kind of expansive joy that I had no idea existed beforehand. And there is no question that this had profound and positive effects on the way I interacted with people and the world. So I know that the idea of the 'discipline' of meditation, twice a day, for a period of many years is just an idea – it is not how it is. I meditated every day, twice a day for seven years, with no problem doing so even when I was travelling. Even on a coach or a train I could easily sit quietly and go to deep, expansive and relaxing spaces.

Vipassana is another powerful meditation technique that many of my friends have explored with significant and extremely positive results. My observation of others is that Vipassana works very well as a way of reaching some very deep levels of experience, moving through some big internal challenges, gaining profound insights and definitely helping to change your life for the better. Following it up after the initial retreat requires a commitment of time (one to two hours a day) – everyone I know who has kept this up says it has paid them huge dividends. The philosophy of the Vipassana movement is definitely something to be admired, as those doing a retreat need not pay, but are encouraged to make a donation according to the value they feel they have received or to work as helpers on future retreats.

Through many friends I also know that breathing and body conscious Buddhist and yoga meditations are also very clarifying and stabilising, and are used by many to great effect. Martial arts related meditations and dynamic meditations such as Tai Chi can also be very powerful. Allowing the mind to follow the breath or the sensations of the body takes it out of its mental sphere – which is the primary objective of meditation. In effect meditation seems to hypnotise the left brain, allowing the powerful right brain out to open up and be more fully and directly experienced, providing its insights and wholly different types of experience to those that dominate our day-to-day life. But understanding how it works is not the important thing... experiencing it, doing it is the important thing.

In reality, once you've got the initial pattern going, and have started to reach some of the deeper states, consistent meditation is usually relatively easy, massively rewarding, and something to look forward to every day rather than to resist.

One of the common themes in meditation teaching is to encourage students not to mix techniques. This is good advice. Various meditation techniques have been developed because they are effective. They work with the nature of the mind to shift us to different beneficial states of being. Thousands of years of observation and practice sit wisely behind most of these techniques. I believe it is worth breaking through our limiting and often somewhat brattish, western ideas of what freedom is. These often emerge in our minds as 'I can do whatever I want; I don't have to do it that way if I don't want to!' My experience is that there is actually far more freedom in finding that we have a choice even within structured practices; I can choose to follow strict guidelines and still be utterly free in that choice. This state of being gives ourselves the opportunity to discover that there are sources and places of freedom that we cannot even imagine. Without feeling we are giving up our freedom, power or control of our lives, we can find that a little 'order' in our lives, and respect for ancient principles, can take us to those places.

The same goes for raw food. I have heard so many times peoples' ideas that it must take so much discipline... it's quite the reverse for me and so many others. In fact, once the first life changes are made, and new patterns established, it is a massive liberation.

Most of these meditation schools do have their own ideas about diet. Most certainly promote vegetarianism and many spiritual schools also combine fasting and meditation for advanced practices. I see natural and complementary benefits in combining more raw foods with meditation practice. My own experience of meditation since going raw is, again, that the clarity that comes from being raw adds another level to the experience. So I feel that any positive change in your lifestyle or diet is likely to deepen your experience of meditation... and vice versa; meditation is only likely to enhance any positive lifestyle or diet changes you make.

Positive Mental and Spiritual Nutrition

At this stage a brief word on positive mental and spiritual nutrition feels important.

I have certainly found it really good for my mental and spiritual health to keep reminding myself to "Programme yourself with positivity, health and sustainability". The media and 'health system' tend to offer a view that disempowers us by telling us it is 'natural' for us to become seriously ill. At times this makes me feel very angry, and at other times very sad, because I believe it is not true, and because I believe many, many human beings experience a huge amount of unnecessary suffering because of this cultural belief in the normality of illness. No one in particular is to blame for this cultural belief, because so many parts of our socio-economic and cultural jigsaw puzzle support and buy into the belief. It's a well established pattern, and a well established belief; it's even a wholly understandable belief... but that does not make it true.

Yes, it is now 'normal' for people to get seriously ill, but it is certainly not natural. And I believe it is not necessary either, given enough information, time, support and confidence in our lives. A little more of a truly scientific and ecological understanding of health, and a stronger, clearer feel for what nature is inside ourselves can help. We all have the potential to move forward from that belief once we have the information and motivation that allows us to replace the old belief with a better informed and more positive new belief.

So to be really effective in changing our own lives for the better we need to close off the taps that keep that negative flow pouring in, and open up the channels that allow a much more positive flow of information and inspiration to flood through our lives. Instead of watching television and buying newspapers that sell the same old drag-me-down messages, change what you feed your mind and spirit on.

It is also useful to recognise that our language and culture is full of restricting or negative subconscious programming. Changing the patterns of words you use, will change the way you think, and changing the way you think will change the way you act. A simple example of this is that we always have a choice to say something other than 'yes' or 'no' – the Japanese have 'yes', 'no' and 'mu', which means something along the lines of 'neither yes nor no; ask a different question!'. So when someone presents me with a narrow 'either/or' choice, I normally find it much more creative and realistic to think of a third option... and often a fourth and fifth too, because I find that nature always offers us much more than just an 'either/or' choice.

To get your positive flow going subscribe to *Permaculture Magazine, The Permaculture Activist, Get FRESH, Living Nutrition, Just Eat An Apple, Positive News,* and other positive publications. Buy a few books that bring you new, positive and helpful information. This will allow you to grow and develop organically. Become part of an active, positive network or some kind of group of friends with a common interest. Explore new activities, be courageous and take the adventurous route that your heart and intuition tell you to. Take some chances, play and explore, mix with and join active, positive networks of people of like mind.

PROGRAMME YOURSELF WITH POSITIVITY, HEALTH AND SUSTAINABILITY

Protesting against the things we don't believe in does still have a positive role. However, I discovered that being mainly 'against' things was part of the clever trap that kept all those negative things dominant in my mind; it gave me no space to create the positive alternatives. We have to shift the majority of our attention and action to creating those positive alternatives, otherwise they will never happen. The personal politics of creation that will naturally lead us to creating more positive, naturally healthy and sustainable lives, and therefore a more positive, naturally healthy and sustainable world, involves getting the balance right – up to one third of our energy can go into protest against what needs changing, at the same time we must ensure that at least two thirds of our action, thoughts and energy and that includes our work, is going into creating the life and the world that we want, deserve and feel is needed for ourselves and future generations. No one else is going to do it for you (or us); we have to create it ourselves.

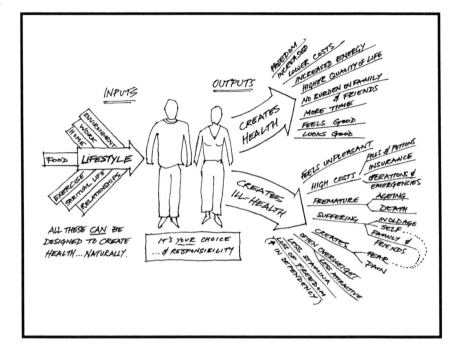

The main suggestion overall is to 'Take Responsibility For Yourself'. Recognise your own power in any and every situation. You have the power of your own will and you have the power to act positively. Use mind-mapping and other tools to explore what you are doing in your life, and where you're heading. Recognise that you have changed, you are changing and you will change. Then identify and take the practical next steps that will change your life positively. And then regularly use mind-mapping and other tools for a period of weeks or a month to plan and implement your own positive and effective personal revolution! Take steps towards a more sustainable and fulfilling life style. This means getting on and doing it. Book yourself on a permaculture course and raw food workshop – go on, you've got nothing to loose and everything to gain. Buy some 'radical reading', books that will change you life.

If you are in a relationship doing this exploration just with your partner can be tremendously creative. However, I also believe that we can get even more out of the process by entering into the adventure of life change with a wider group of friends. So preferably do all or some of your exploration on your own, or with your partner, and also do it with friends and/or family to discover new ways of doing things, that provide mutual support and fun.

Just reading about these steps to change your life will have some small effect. And taking one or two steps as a result will create a little ripple effect of change. Taking at least four or five steps will really start things moving positively though!

Holistic Eco-Health

Meditation is like a form of massage or yoga for the mind and spirit. The physical equivalent is equally important for complete health, for 'a new holistic eco-health...' Physical exercise and body movement is required for excellent heath. In particular it helps our breathing and as 60% of our energy is said to come from the air we breathe (via the burning of oxygen in our cells) this is very important. This is one of the reasons why physically active people on a poor diet can maintain excellent health... until they become less active, when the effects of their diet then become proportionately much more of an influence, and often very suddenly they then become ill.

My short list of suggestions as to what you could select for physical exercise includes: Yoga, The Five Tibetans[51], Tai Chi, Aikido ('The Way of Peace', particularly the Ki school), dancing, and for the more physical and 'sporty' surprisingly enough the Royal Canadian Air Force 5BX programme, which is designed to get pilots to peak fitness with just 11 minutes of very carefully designed exercise per day[52].

This is an area in my own life where I have not been consistent and that I know still needs attention for me to achieve a more complete state of health. However, I have practiced Tai Chi and the Five Tibetans for extended periods with very significant effects. In the past playing a lot of sport, plus plenty of cycling and walking (which I still do plenty of) have kept me generally fit. I have dabbled enough with the 5BX programme to know that it can generate high levels of fitness in a very short space of time.

For a more complete health, and particularly if you live in a town or city, I feel it can be very important to reduce or remove the often consistent underlying stresses and tensions about fear of physical attack. Personally, I have sensed for a long time that in a world which we are told is 'dangerous', and where we are told to constantly fear attack and physical violence, that learning some form of self-defence (physical and psychological) can help bring greater freedom into our lives, by creating a feeling of greater self-confidence. It may seem strange, but it is true that for me going raw has strengthened my psychological confidence because I feel immune to the fear of attack from the normal humdrum illnesses. But, on the physical defence front I still need to build my confidence, as many of us do.

At the time of writing I am just starting to explore the world of Aikido – 'The Way of Peace'. And I can see that contrary to my old ideas of macho martial arts, the Ki school of Aikido emphasises nature, peace and harmony, as well as giving and mutual benefit. The recent dramatic and powerfully energising and centering effect it has had on a good friend of mine has been immediately

---

[51] See the small and fascinating book *The Five Tibetans*, Christopher Kilham, Healing Arts Press, 1994 – also *Just Eat An Apple*, Jan – Feb 2001 edition (issue 15) for an excellent summary by Frederic Paténaude.

[52] See the small, neat book *The Royal Canadian Air Force 5BX Programme*.

noticeable. We need power but not aggression to change our lives for the better with confidence. I sense that Aikido and other spiritually based martial arts are powerful and effective parts of the personal web-of-health that we need to spin in our lives to make more of our full potential, bringing more confidence and straight-forward positive action, as well as more health and joy into our lives.

I know from my own life it can be hard to keep all the plates spinning all of the time; to juggle the various balls in one's life and keep them going all together. It's a great challenge to try to spin the complete web, and I can see and feel how amazing it will be when I do bring all the parts of the jigsaw together in my own life. Personally I sense that my own centering, energizing six-fold power-pack of personal lifestyle permaculture will include:

* Raw food (vegan).

* Meditation.

* Yoga, The Five Tibetans, Tai chi or Aikido.

* (Vegan) Permaculture, Forest/Paradise Gardening.

* Expressive, artistic, creative endeavours, such as music, singing, writing, performance, painting, etc.

* Living in a positive community situation, and/or working/being with a group of friends who are learning, working and walking together in a parallel positive direction, like an extended family, or a 'tribe' – for me this is my life at Ecoforest, and my work with other friends and networks.

I am not there yet. I haven't got the whole package in place, although I have explored several of these elements in isolation, and in combination with several others. On an increasing number of days I have even managed four and sometimes five of the six at the same time! These explorations have all had positive effects on my life in themselves. So I am hoping to share knowledge and enthusiasm, and do not need to give myself a hard time for 'not being perfect', or for not bringing all these elements together at the same time in my life yet. I have made choices about my priorities, and they have probably been right for the time and the place. Having said that, I know that bringing these things together at the same time will have a massively powerful and positive effect. There will be no turning back – only going forward. So why not consider taking that step... and do so with a big smile on your face! Let me know how you get on.

There is a bit of a pattern with these very significant life changes. It is not always a matter of a linear progression from one step to the next, as one step can lead to several others happening at the same time. What I see is a beautiful spider's web, with different segments relating to Earth Care, People Care and Fair Shares. Each segment is connected by any number of finely spun strands.

You can enter into the web from any number of the anchoring strands that connect it to the world that it is part of. Imagine such a web for yourself...

imagine where you might choose to enter, and what strands to your web you might have.

For example, you might find that a general and gradually rising concern for the environment might lead you to take the positive step of doing a full permaculture course. This might then raise your understanding of the interconnectedness of Earth Care – People Care – Fair Share issues, which then leads you to choose to change your food buying and eating habits, for both ethical and intellectual reasons. And then you might find that you realise that diet, personal health and ecological issues are intimately linked... which leads you to vegetarianism, veganism or raw food; or may be to doubling the amount of 'raw' in your life, and halving or cutting out the milk, meat 'n' wheat if that is still part of your life.

With these changes you might then discover it doesn't feel like you thought it would. In fact it feels easy. And rather than feeling like a denial of something it feels like a positive and liberating choice. This then opens new doors for you... which you stride through with greater confidence. It leads you to more people care; a greater sense of understanding and empathy with yourself and with others; which again feels good. So with a confident spring in your step and a gentle smile on your face you then start off down the personal development pathway. This in turn leads you to still more self-confidence; more confidence to explore and experiment with life-change, and a letting go of old blockages about what 'spiritual' means. So then you might find that you choose freely to start to meditate... Just take some time and imagine a little longer...

All these life changes add up, and they can happen one by one, or in a cluster. What is clear is that they create very signifcantly different and more positive effects in the 'outside' world, as a reflection of the changes that have happened in the inner world.

The reality is that you can choose to start along a path of positive life change by passing through any one of these 'doorways'. Any one of them can lead you to other areas of discovery and growth. One initial change, like a stone thrown in a pond, has a ripple effect which changes your thinking and behaviour in other areas.

For me meditation was the doorway into all the other areas of concern – where some doors were ajar, suddenly they started flying open. This led to a raised level of general awareness, that naturally allowed my underlying interest in nature to grow into fully blown environmental concern; so an eco-spiritual seed was sown, a seed that has grown strongly ever since. My gradually opening eyes led me to do a full permaculture course, where by chance I met a knowledgbable raw fooder, who had already been raw for two and a half years. And being an ecologically minded vegan already that got me into the raw food thing. In turn all these things have led me to want to create an ecological community that suits me, with others that I know have similar views, interests, concerns and visions. And that has created a place, which is now my home, called Ecoforest.

The spider's web we each weave is in effect our own personal 'web of life'.

Each web has segments; one each for your shopping patterns, diet, exercise, meditation, food growing and so on. And you may have some parts of your web complete in your life (say 2 or 3 out of 6 or 7 sections), or you may have the whole thing complete. The web is connected to a whole chain of strands that are anchored to various effects in the outside world, and the inside world of mind, body, emotions and spirit. So there's an Earth Care – People Care – Fair Share web of internal and external effects. And the web of internal effects is parallel to and connected to the web of external effects. All these aspects of your life you can design to be mutually beneficial as part of your 'personal permaculture plan' to redesign or to fine tune your life.

So if you want to change the world, you have to starting changing and respinning your own web of life.

The Role of Permaculture

Permaculture can empower us all to take greater control of our food production, and our lives in general. It can help increase the personal and planetary benefits of growing and eating our food. It takes a whole lot of things – self seeding plants, perennial vegetables, fruiting trees and shrubs, herbs, companion planting, compost heaps, ponds, ground cover plants, climbers, water use, waste, appropriate technology, ecological building and much more too. It gives you the power to make your own recipe of combinations in life that suit you. Whether you have a window sill or balcony, or a thousand acre farm, permaculture can help you get more out from putting less in – and in a much more planet friendly way.

Permaculture offers real opportunities to create much more sustainable lifestyles and living environments in urban, semi-urban and rural situations. Beyond that I am only now starting to grasp the full implications of the use of permaculture thinking in designing our physical, mental, emotional and spiritual nutrition, health and personal development.

Working with nature involves generating a sense of oneness – feel like a tree; think like a pond; see the world from a bramble's perspective! See the whole system that you are part of as your extended family; trees, herbs, insects and wildlife – feel that all these are your parents, grandparents, sisters, brothers, cousins, aunts and uncles. All working together for the good of the family, all caring for each other and providing for each other's needs, through living, loving relationships. We all share the same life-force, and ultimately we are all made of the same stuff. This kind of enjoyable and useful altered perspective is one kind of thinking that permaculture points us towards. But it is not a 'fluffy' perspective – it's only when you get a real and connected feel or vision of nature's abundance and creativity that you can start to really work with her power and wisdom to create true health and sustainability.

And that's not all, because permaculture can also be used in a very scientific, or engineering minded, way too – and to great effect. In fact a scientific approach to permaculture thinking has massive potential. The key is to wake up scientifically minded people and engineers to that fact...

Various permaculture books are useful in gaining more insight into permaculture theory and practice. In particular the following will help to shed light on the various topics in this section: *Introduction to Permaculture* (by Bill Mollison et al); *Forest Gardening* (by Robert Hart); *The Permaculture Garden* (by Graham Bell); *The Earth Care Manual, How To Make A Forest Garden* and *Permaculture In A Nutshell* (by Patrick Whitefield) and *Plants For A Future* (by Ken Fern). If you buy, read and use any three or more of these books you'll be well on your way.[53]

Permaculture Magazine, published by Permanent Publications (UK), is also indispensable and not only for temperate climates and the UK, whilst *The Permaculture Activist* (USA) is a great voice for permaculture in north America. The very best thing to do is to buy yourself a copy of one of these magazines, go to the courses section at the back (or visit the Permaculture Association website or one of the sites listed on page 159) and book yourself on a permaculture course right away! Simple.

Learning About Permaculture: Zones, Sectors and Slope

Considering 'zones, sectors and slope' in permaculture is about efficient energy planning. It is all about efficient use of the energy that is stored in and which flows through the site.

Permaculture usually uses ZONES as a flexible tool to design for maximum efficiency in the work we do, in planting and so on – maximum output with minimum unnecessary effort.

The dwelling (or other building, such as a school) is seen as Zone 0, with Zone 1 immediately around the house. We then move out through the other zones to Zone 5 which is always included, for some wilderness which is just left for nature to play with.

Zones 1 and 2 are the intensive gardening zones. Zone 1 is mainly for all-year salad and herb cultivation, with the plants that need most attention and energy input, and the plants that will be picked from virtually every day, as well as wall climbers, small shrubs, a pond (however small) and maybe some dwarf trees or trained trees on the wall, a fence or some other vertical element. Rainwater collection and a compost heap are also common Zone 1 elements. Zone 2 is for other vegetables, soft fruit and fruit trees that need less energy input and attention, making it the main forest gardening or food forest zone. Zone 3 is the commercial and extensive agriculture or agroforestry zone, and Zone 4 is for managed woodland and forest. Zone 5 is for wilderness; a space for nature and wildlife to do as it wishes.

So you can see that this is a flexible system, as you probably won't have many trees for timber growing in your suburban garden or the backyard of your terraced house! Ponds are particularly valuable in Zones 1 and 2, as are

---

[53] Available from Permanent Publications by mail order or may be ordered online at their website: www.permaculture.co.uk

climbers – whether they are grape vines, sugar snap peas, runner beans, passion fruit, Siberian kiwi or brambles.

The point with zoning is that it helps structure your thinking during the design stage. So, as an example, it means that unlike the traditional garden you don't put most of the veg garden and compost heap hidden away at the bottom of a long garden plot, where you can't see what is really going on unless you're there and which you don't want to trudge down to on a wet and windy autumn or winter afternoon. Instead you put your salads, herbs, veg, soft fruit and compost system much closer, where they will naturally get more and better attention – which will normally automatically mean it is more productive. And you can easily integrate some flowers in with the veg bed both for their own beauty, because many are delicious to eat and for their benefits with pollination and for attracting pest predator insects.

Zoning can also be considered beyond the house and plot. Zones A to G cover:

A) The house and grounds (Zones 0-5).

B) The immediate environment, neighbourhood or local settlement.

C) The district/town (or municipality).

D) The bio-region.

E) The country as a whole.

F) The global region (e.g. Europe, or north America).

G) The Earth, the globe, the living planet as a whole – so G is for Gaia.

The practicalities of sustainable lifestyle design with Zones A to G are:

* Zone A: (Zones 0-5): aim for *at least* 50% of needs to be met within this zone.

* Zone B: neighbourhood/community: at least 75% of needs from Zones B + A.

* Zone C: municipality: at least 87% of needs (A-C).

* Zone D: Bioregion: at least 93% of needs (A-D).

* Zone E: Nation (or state in US/Canada /Aus, etc.): at least 96% of needs (A-E).

* Zone F: Global region (e.g. Western Europe): at least 98% of needs (A-F).

* Zone G: Gaia, the globe, the planet as a whole: at least 99% of needs (A-G).

* Which leaves the possibility of up to 1% of needs being met from cosmic sources of supply!

In teaching 2 week permaculture courses and 2 day 'introduction to permaculture' courses I find this a really helpful model that gives people a sense of context, for their life 'outside' and for the more well known Zones 0-5. It gives Zones 0 to 5 a connection with the locality, the bioregion and beyond, so that people can see the local-to-global picture as a whole.

This is a very flexible model and needs to be stressed as just a rough guide. However, after years of work on local to national sustainability projects and Agenda 21, as well as grassroots permaculture I feel that the guide figures for the proportion of your needs to be met from within each band of Zones are

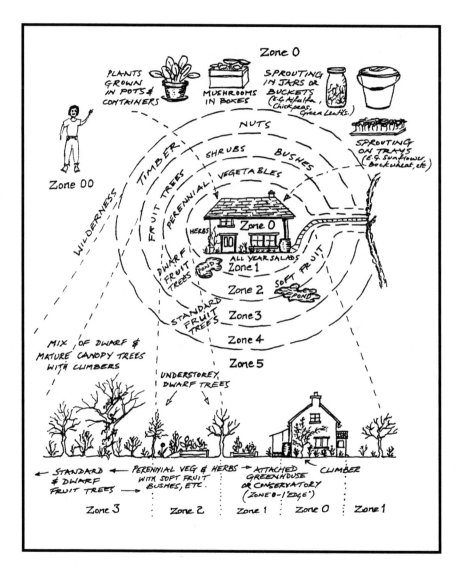

Zone 0

PLANTS GROWN IN POTS & CONTAINERS

MUSHROOMS IN BOXES

SPROUTING IN JARS OR BUCKETS (E.G. Alfalfa, Chickpeas, Green Lentils.)

SPROUTING ON TRAYS (E.G. Sunflower, Buckwheat, etc)

Zone 00

WILDERNESS
TIMBER
FRUIT TREES
SHRUBS
BUSHES
NUTS
PERENNIAL
VEGETABLES
HERBS
DWARF FRUIT TREES
ALL YEAR SALADS
SOFT FRUIT
STANDARD FRUIT TREES

Zone 0

POND

Zone 1

Zone 2

POND

Zone 3

Zone 4

Zone 5

MIX OF DWARF & MATURE CANOPY TREES WITH CLIMBERS

UNDERSTOREY, DWARF TREES

← STANDARD & DWARF FRUIT TREES →

← PERENNIAL VEG & HERBS WITH SOFT FRUIT BUSHES, ETC.

→ ATTACHED GREENHOUSE OR CONSERVATORY (ZONE 0-1 'EDGE')

CLIMBER

Zone 3

Zone 2

Zone 1

Zone 0

Zone 1

very practical, relatively easy to understand and very handy – halving what's left each time. It works very well as a practical guide for people wanting to look at how to transform their impacts by focusing on how they meet their needs – or more simply, how and where they spend their energy and money.[54]

Basically, if the bioregional level is sorted most of the rest is. In other words, as a guide, if you meet 93% or more of your needs from within the BioRegion you will be living a pretty sustainable life. In my permaculture course session on BioRegions I expand on this and discuss the types of needs that are most likely to be met within certain zones. This helps to get across that we are not talking just about physical needs. Most of our physical needs can and should be met within the bioregional zone, and particularly the more local zones. So, for example, food needs in particular would aim to be met primarily from Zones A to C, as would a lot of social needs. Construction needs would primarily be met from Zones A to C as well, although a certain proportion of materials could come from wider areas of the bioregion. Until very recently building needs were always met at the bioregional level, and led to regionally distinct and therefore much more interesting styles of houses and other buildings. It is one area that we could relatively easily shift to sustainability, both in the design and the performance of buildings if we allowed our thinking to evolve, in line with many of the excellent examples of ecological design and building that already exist[55]. Needs for information, networks, a great deal of research and so on are another area that are very well met at the bioregional level.

So thinking in terms of these zones can really help to change your consumer impacts in a very significant and positive way.

Thinking about diet runs from Zone G down has Zone oo – the one zone not yet mentioned; Zone oo is the person. Diet has huge implications for so many aspects of your lifestyle. In permaculture terms it effects all our living space from Zones o (inside the house) to 5 (the wildlife or wilderness area), taking in all our food growing areas (Zones 1 to 4) in between. It also has much wider implications in Zones A to G.

For example, humanity's use of just five crops – wheat, maize, rice, soya and potatoes – to supply more than 50% of its global food consumption is directly linked to the typical diets people eat. All these mono-crops, apart from maize (which is deeeee-licious raw), need to be cooked. If you change what you eat and how you obtain it, you change a lot. So it's the inter-connected chain of effects in all these zones, from Zone oo to Zone 5, and from Zone A to Zone G that I am asking you to think about... and then to intelligently design some positive changes to benefit yourself, others and nature/the earth.

The permaculture of diet is essentially a matter of designing the designer. As all design comes from the designer (Zone oo) it seems particularly sensible to

---

[54] If I had time I'd check the model out in relation to Wakenagel et al's excellent 'Ecological Footprint' work! See their book if you are interested and want more information.

[55] See www.sustainablehousing.org.uk if you are particularly interested in sustainable construction issues.

design for health and productivity in that part of the overall system. 'Holistic eco-health' is about design for Zone oo.

SECTORS are about looking at how energy flows through and within your site – the sunny sectors of your site and the shady areas, the winter sunrise and sunset, and the summer sunrise and sunset; about the prevailing wind, any dominant cold winds – the windy and sheltered sectors; and about any water that flows or stands in your site – the wet and the dry sectors, and fire risk sectors in warmer climates. It's about how you place plants and other elements in the landscape to make the most of the sun, shelter, water and so on. It's about how natural energy moves in your site and how you can influence that – including the energies of human movement, wind and water flow and plant growth.

In many senses we can also see times of day and seasons of the year as sectors in time. During each day we go through various cycles. So for example morning may be one kind of sector and the evening another; the same can be said of summer and winter. In terms of diet, for me this has meant I have a slightly different balance of raw foods depending on what sector of the day and year I am in; with heavier foods such as nuts in winter and lighter fruit in summer... following nature's patterns.

Permaculture also looks at how SLOPES can be used to best advantage – slopes that face the sun, what grows well on a cooler, shaded slope, sheltered spots, where the frost pockets lie, and how slopes can be used to reduce work by planting timber and self seeding trees, such as oak or nut trees, at the top of the slope. On a smaller scale this works well with self-seeding salad plants, and in both cases the action of gravity, often aided by the movement of water, moves the seeds down the slope, spreading them down and across the slope over time. In particular slope is vital for using and moving water for maximum benefit, and with the least work – and in permaculture this means understanding that movements of water below the ground surface on a slope are at least as important as those above the surface.

When you start to overlay the zones, sectors and slopes you will really see how many microclimates you have on your site. In this way you can see which combinations of zones, sectors and slopes work together to create good conditions, and which work to create much tougher conditions. This way you can design in uses, plants, water features, waste and water management systems, and so on that are best suited to the various niches that are available.

In your Zone oo 'personal permaculture plan' you can consider slopes as being motivations, with positive motivations being like a down hill slope that help you move forward. Resistances, blockages and ruts in your life can be like up-hill slopes and dark or sunken areas – they can be turned to something positive and productive but they require careful design to do so. When adapting this tool in this way to looking at your own life as a whole, Zones 1 and 2 are the areas of your life into which you put most energy, and which therefore hopefully are most productive for you – if they are not it is time for some redesign of your life! Sectors are where you have energy coming in from the outside, which might be information, skills, money or friendship. Thinking about your life in this way, doing your own 'personal permaculture plan' for Zone oo, and applying permaculture design principles to the flows of energy, patterns and different zones of your life can be incredibly useful and enjoyable, as well as hugely productive!

Perennials, Self - Seeders, Companions and Guilds

Perennials and self-seeders are a vital part of permaculture because once started, unlike annual crops, they require little or no work to produce a harvest. Perennials include trees, shrubs and bushes, as well as perennial vegetables and herbs. For those concerned with nutrition perennials are particularly important because they maintain and provide high mineral and nutrient levels which are much closer to natural wild foods than the highly manipulated annual vegetable strains. The later section on forest gardens shows how a whole, low maintenance food producing system can be designed with perennials of all types forming the foundations of that system.

The permaculture movement in general, and the Plants For A Future project in particular, have created a huge and tremendously useful resource of information on perennial vegetable and salad plants, and the many uses of various herbs, shrubs and trees – a resource that is now easily accessible via books and the internet.

Get into pick'n'pluck and cut'n'come vegetables and salad leaves – they provide easy and useful contributions to the diet. Cut'n'come again plants, for example, actually grow more when some of their leaves are harvested (e.g. chives, corn salad, rocket, spinach, pak choi, mizuna, radish, rape leaf, cabbage, land cress, leaf celery, lemon balm, red-leaved chicory, mint, parsley, coriander, endive, claytonia, purslane, etc.). A note on radish is that if you allow it to set seed, and harvest many of the young pods for food you will get much more food from the plant than if you harvest its leaves or root. This also allows the plant its full life cycle and ensures an abundant supply of radish when the seed germinates.

Use pick'n'pluck vegetables. These include spinach beet, Swiss chard, sorrel, perennial broccoli, watercress, fennel, seakale, tree onions, Welsh onions and everlasting onions, garlic, horseradish, broad beans, courgette, angelica, lovage, sweet cicely, and so on.

Companion plants are plants that grow well together. Examples of good companions are tomatoes and marigolds. These should be used as well as and alongside GUILDS. A guild takes this idea further by creating groupings of plants that work well together. A guild is where the whole is greater than the sum of its parts. The classic example of a guild is the native American combination of beans, maize and squash – a sacred combination called 'the Three Sisters'. The beans fix nitrogen and grow up the maize, while the squash produces a living mulch and they all produce a crop of course, whilst meeting each others basic needs without the need for external inputs. A classic north wall guild in the UK is morello cherry, with alpine strawberries, red currents, gooseberries or the very elegant and easily propagated Japanese wineberry.

In nutritional terms, a good balance of vitamins, minerals and food enzymes is a guild, because you obtain more nutritional value from foods which contain all of these. Having green leafy veg with either protein foods or starch foods is more of a 'companion food' than a nutritional guild. A guild is a consciously designed grouping that creates a combination and a whole effect that is greater and more positive than just the sum of its parts. It's like multiplying a group of numbers together, rather than adding them.[56]

A Summary of Permaculture Design Principles

There is a nice progression from 3 to 6 to 12 in the core permaculture ethics and principles. You don't need to remember them all, you just need to remember to use them and that they are here in this book whenever you need them. And when you start to use them in your life you will find that you naturally remember a useful number of them.

The 3 Ethics

1. **Earth Care:** looking after the planet's needs, and the local ecology.

2. **People Care:** looking after human needs – physical, social, psychological.

3. **Fair Share:** for people and planet, limits to consumption and sharing surplus.

The 6 Attitudinal Principles

1. **The Problem Is The Solution:** turn problems to solutions and liabilities to assets.

2. **Maximum Output for Minimum Effort:** the effect should be greater than effort; increased output greater than input.

3. **The Yield Is Theoretically Unlimited:** increase the total yields: small changes can notch up yield in subtle ways, and see/create gardens as ecosystems.

4. **Work With Nature:** nature knows best: learn from and work with nature, not against it, outside and inside.

5. **Everything Gardens:** everything works to create the environment it needs; every element has some effect in the system, so make the effects positive.

6. **Harvest Only Sunshine:** use only renewable resources, and be positive in your thoughts and actions. Create 'closed loop' systems.

The 12 Technical Design Principles

1. **Relative location:** think about how one thing is placed in relation to others, so that elements meet each others needs and use each others outputs.

2. **Multi-use:** make sure every element you design in is multi-functional, with at least 3 uses.

---

[56] Assuming those numbers are all greater than one!

3. **Multi-supply:** meet each need from a variety of sources... 'don't put all your eggs in one basket'.

4. **Energy efficient planning: zones, sectors and slope.**

5. **Accelerated succession:** speed up nature's natural processes of growth, fertility building and diversity.

6. **Cycling of energy and resources:** the more you cycle energy and resources within your system the more productive it will be, with less effort.

7. **Biological resources:** what you use to meet your needs and the needs of your 'pc system' should be biological where ever possible.

8. **Diversity:** follow the pattern of nature, which is diversity = multi-function, multi-supply, stability and productivity.

9. **Small scale intensive systems:** these systems are most productive, 'start at your backdoor and work out on a controlled front'.

10. **Edge effect:** the edge between ecosystems (like the pond or woodland edge) is often most productive – use this effect, create lots of 'edge' to raise your own productivity.

11. **Appropriate technology:** use technology that is environmentally and culturally appropriate, which is easily maintained, affordable and repairable.

12. **Stacking in space and time:** use vertical space and create systems which give a harvest throughout the year.

Three useful permaculture 'soundbites':

✳ "Unused outputs = pollution" i.e. you need to 'work' to remove any output that is not used by another element of the system.

✳ "Unmet needs = work" i.e. you need to work to meet any needs of an element that are not met by the output of another element.

✳ "No bare soil" i.e. any plant, even a 'weed', helps to protect the soil from sun and rain, and to build up the life and fertility of the soil, so no space should be left with bare soil. For good reason, nature does not leave soil bare.

The Design Process

There is no single permaculture design process; rather there are a selection of tools and techniques, tricks and checklists that you can use to guide the design and implementation process. For example, as well as considering 'zone, sector and slope' you can adopt the multi-functional 'Three-Use Rule' which suggests that all elements in a designed or adapted system should have at least three uses or benefits. For example, a simple hedge can provide food, shelter from the wind for plants and people, beauty and a wildlife habitat, as well as being a boundary marker and a barrier to keep larger animals out. A pond can provide food, relaxation and beauty, a wildlife habitat and home for slug-munching frogs, and if it is carefully placed it can also reflect extra solar radiation into a conservatory or greenhouse in the winter. A cycle path network can create a sustainable transport and wildlife corridor, be an element in a public health strategy and community art strategy with sculptures lining the route, an education resource, and could also be planted to produce food.

Another useful tool is the OBREDIM checklist that guides you through the design process:

The OBREDIM Design Stages

O **Objectives and Observation:** for and of the site, its users, its surroundings, the energy flowing through it, and so on. Get your objective clear first, then just stick to observation if you can, note down thoughts, try to leave the designing until later.

B **Boundaries and Resources** – recording and mapping them. Walk the boundaries and look into the site, and away from it. Record onsite resources and those available nearby.

R **Research**

E **Evaluation and examination** – of site data and other information; putting a 'value' to the things being considered in terms of their capacity to help you achieve the objectives of your design.

D **Design** – placing things together and creating the relationships between elements and flows that will enable you to achieve your design objectives.

I **Implementation** – including design phasing of implementation, and planning what resources you will need to use and when.

M **Monitoring, Modification and Maintenance** – Get a feel for or look at how well your systems are working and make adjustments (to either the system or your objectives – or both) as necessary.

Wild design is another approach to design that can use free brain storming or some other process that consciously uses creative chaos as a catalyst for ideas and inspiration. Wild design is then followed by a consideration of what useful and creative ideas have appeared. The design process is important in permaculture. There is no 'right' way to do it, but the tools above and a range of others will always help you to get more out of your design with less hard work – both during the design, as well as in the implementation and maintenance phases. And one of your main design objectives might be to create a really good, low maintenance forest garden system...

What is Forest Gardening?

Forest gardening involves the creation of a productive and stable mini-forest, that is packed full of food producing plants, shrubs and trees. The forest garden concept is rooted in an understanding of forest ecology, so

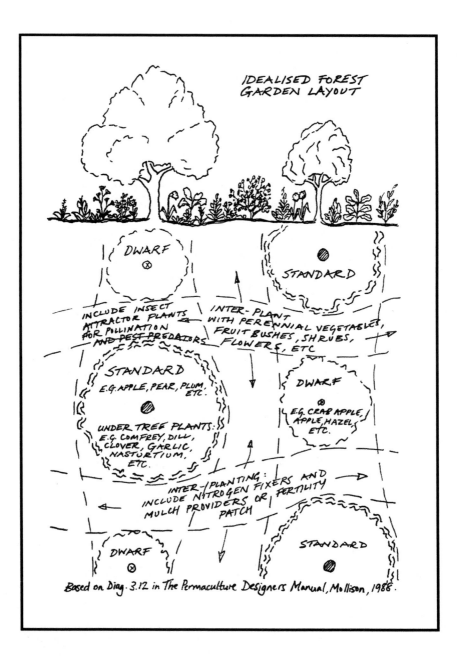

IDEALISED FOREST GARDEN LAYOUT

DWARF ⊗

STANDARD ●

INCLUDE INSECT ATTRACTOR PLANTS FOR POLLINATION AND PEST PREDATORS

INTER-PLANT WITH PERENNIAL VEGETABLES, FRUIT BUSHES, SHRUBS, FLOWERS, ETC

STANDARD
E.G. APPLE, PEAR, PLUM, ETC.
●

UNDER TREE PLANTS:
E.G. COMFREY, DILL, CLOVER, GARLIC, NASTURTIUM, ETC.

DWARF
E.G. CRAB APPLE, APPLE, HAZEL, ETC.

INTER-PLANTING: INCLUDE NITROGEN FIXERS AND MULCH PROVIDERS OR FERTILITY PATCH

DWARF ⊗

STANDARD ●

Based on Diag. 3.12 in The Permaculture Designers Manual, Mollison, 1988.

in particular it works with the different layers of a forest system and places together plants that benefit each other. The forest garden is one of the most useful, most effective and most widely used ideas in permaculture, because it is quite simple to understand. The forest garden aims to create and use up to seven layers in a garden or growing system. These seven layers are: the canopy, smaller trees (often shade tolerant), shrubs, herbaceous, ground cover, roots and climbers. The fundamental objective is to make every layer productive and useful, and to create positive, beneficial relationships amongst plants and creatures within and between each layer. As Robert Hart, the 'inventor' of the forest garden in Britain, says:

"Diversity is the keynote of the forest garden concept, but it must be an ordered diversity, governed by the principles and laws of plant symbiosis; all plants must be compatible with each other. Most forest gardens are designed primarily to meet the needs of the cultivators and their families for food, fuel, fibres, timber and other necessities, but some can also include a cash component.

The forest garden is the most productive of all forms of land use... [It] is far more than a system for supplying mankind's material needs. It is a way of life that also supplies people's spiritual needs by its beauty and the wealth of wildlife it attracts." [57]

The British permaculture designer, teacher and author Patrick Whitefield prefers the term 'woodland garden' as he feels this is easier to relate to the British situation. A woodland tends to imply something more diverse and natural than our ideas of forests. However, whilst making this useful point, Patrick also feels that because the term 'forest garden' has become widely used it is easier to stick with that.[58] In Australia and some other areas the term 'food forest' is also used – so use which ever term you like best!

"Whilst the cultivation of conventional vegetables involves the arduous and fiddlesome annual chores of digging, raking, preparing seed-beds, sowing, transplanting, thinning out, hoeing, weeding, watering and composting, the herbs and perennial vegetables are quite happy to look after themselves. They need little or no watering or composting, because their deep roots draw up water and minerals from the subsoil, for the benefit of themselves and each other, and they don't even need weeding or hoeing, as they quickly spread over the whole surface of the soil, suppressing all competitors, while their intricate tangle of roots maintain a porous soil-structure." Robert Hart.[59]

Forest gardening embodies the key permaculture principle of STACKING. This involves using vertical space to its full extent, so that every level of the garden, from ground to canopy, are productive. Time Stacking is also used to plan for a harvest throughout the year – both these elements of stacking are indicated in the table of potential forest garden species, see Appendix 4.

---

[57] From *Forest Gardening*, by Robert Hart, Green Books, Hartland, 1991.

[58] From *How To Make A Forest Garden* by Patrick Whitefield, Permanent Publications, 1996.

[59] From *The Forest Garden*, Inst. for Social Inventions, Third Edition, 1992.

SEVEN STOREYS OF TEMPERATE FOREST GARDEN

1. CANOPY (Largest Fruit Trees: standards, etc.)
2. LOW TREE LAYER (Dwarfing stock, shade tolerant, etc.)
3. SHRUBS (Currants, Berries, etc.)
4. HERBACEOUS (Herbs, Perenial Veg, etc.)
5. VERTICAL (Climbers, Vines, etc.)
6. GROUND COVER (Strawberries, Dewberries, creeping Herbs, etc.)
7. ROOT CROPS (Vegetables, Tubers, etc.)

The Forest Garden mimics the natural, therefore sustainable, forest ecosystem. It requires minimum maintenance, and it maximizes output, because it uses plants that naturally benefit each other — companion plants & 'guilds'.

MULCHING is a key technique that is widely used in forest gardening and most other permacultures, because is has so many benefits. This involves putting a thick layer of organic material over the soil, around plants, newly planted trees and trees that are already established,[60] and planting new plants and trees into or through the mulch layer. Mulching protects the soil from excessive heat and cold, as well as from wind and rain, and keeps the soil moist in summer. It prevents and discourages unwanted plants from competing with those that have been planted, which is particularly important for young trees. It adds to the fertility of the soil by allowing organic matter to break down and be taken into the soil, thereby helping it to develop and release its own natural fertility without digging. If you compare any mulched soil with the soil in any non-organic arable field, you will find that the former is teeming with the life that allows it to build and release its fertility, while the latter is a largely dead soil which requires significant inputs to allow crops to be grown commercially. The idea of ground cover plants is that they create a living mulch. And the general intention in a permaculture design is to fill or cover every area of soil, either with plants or with mulch.

It is worth being aware that in warmer climates, and in developing countries in particular, forest gardening is both particularly effective, and often familiar. In such climates, and in more severe situations, once established forest gardens help to protect sensitive plants from intensive sun and wind, preventing soil erosion, promoting water retention and therefore the build up of available groundwater, increasing fertility, and also providing many crops of course. Wherever you are, if some water is available then forest gardens can be planted and established even in very marginal sites or regions. There are at least 30 food producing species of tree that will even grow in a desert situation. As plant-based food systems, forest gardening and agroforestry are the most practical solution in many of the ecologically degraded and desertified regions of the world – and quite possibly the only practical solution, both in terms of ecological regeneration and sustainable food production.

In terms of what is practical for you, once you have a basic layout established and probably some trees and/or bushes in place, establishing your winter salads is a particularly useful project to start on in a permaculture design or a forest garden – then work on the spring and early summer salads. It is also possible to add fungi into your forest garden system, such as shitake mushrooms.

The following will also help to increase the yield and health of the whole system, whether it is a forest garden or any other permaculture system:

✳ Nitrogen fixers: e.g. in temperate systems *Eleagnus*, clover, lucerne/alfalfa, beans, alder, black locust/false acacia, Siberian pea tree, etc. In sub-tropical/ Mediterranean climates: tagasaste, leucaena, albizia, beans, peas, lucernce/ alfalfa, etc.

---

[60] Mulch should be spread up to a metre around trees, say 10cm deep, leaving a space of about 10cm around the trunk of the tree.

* Mulch plants: e.g. reeds (*Phragmites australis/communis*), aromatic herbs to deter slugs (mints, tansy, balm, etc). Oak leaf mould is also a good slug deterrent.

* Pest repellents: e.g. onion/allium family (chive, garlic, etc.), marigolds, etc.

* Green manure/fertility patch: e.g. comfrey, clover, lucerne/alfalfa, buckwheat, chicory, dandelion, nettles, yarrow.

* Insect attractors for pollination: e.g. calendula, borage, chives, buddleia, etc.

* Host plants for predators of pest insects: e.g. chives, buckwheat.

* Species for pollination: e.g. crab apple.

Particularly interesting and powerful foods for the body and brain health can be integrated into any system. Apart from the well known herbs such as thyme, this might include: *Ginkgo biloba* for the brain and circulation improving qualities of its leaves; *Hippophae rhamnoides/salicifolia* for its small but vital fruits that are being researched for use against cancer; and St Johns wort (*Hypericum*) for its beneficial effects on the brain (combined with *Passiflora* it makes an excellent 'happy tea' mix).

Permanent Publications, *Permaculture Magazine* and the associated website www.permaculture.co.uk are superb sources of information for establishing forest gardens and permaculture systems. (see Appendix 3).

The Role of Flowers

Flowers are particularly important in creating a permaculture, and have many uses. The beauty they add to a garden is a vitalising force – beauty is a food for the soul! Apart from their beauty, many flowers are also edible – for example mallow, nasturtiums, milkweeds, calendula, campanulas, yellow asphodel, chives, onions and the day lily.

Flowers are also vitally important for creating a good insect habitat, which is essential for pollination and for a wonderful wildlife garden. So the role and placement of flowers needs careful consideration in its own right within forest garden design.

Wild Foods

Wild foods are the ultimate in cheap and hugely nutritious food – as the title of Richard Mabey's well known book *Food For Free* points out. Wild foods are up to fifty times as mineral rich as vegetables produced by conventional agriculture and horticulture. Franz Konz is particularly well-known in the German natural health movement for promoting the great health benefits of wild foods, whilst David Wolfe and others emphasise their benefits to the English speaking world.

Even in towns and cities, by finding the surprising number of unpolluted and un-fouled places, wild foods can be a simple and nutritious addition to our diet. Dandelions, chickweed, ribbed plantain, lime tree leaves, Jack-by-the -Hedge (or hedge garlic), ransoms (or wild garlic), ground ivy (which has a 'love it', or 'hate it' flavour), nettles[61] and then there's blackberries, chestnuts, hazelnuts and a variety of mushrooms (which need to be identified carefully of course) – all these can make their contribution. *Ginkgo biloba*, mulberries, medlars and other wonderful trees, whilst not wild, are also available in many public parks. And you can of course start to notice wild foods in your own garden, and stop seeing them as 'weeds'.

Eating foods from your climate makes a difference to a raw food body's temperature tolerance. Eating tropical fruit makes the body think it's in a tropical climate. Eating food from your own climate, from your own patch, means the body knows where it's at temperature wise. Also eating food from the place where you live obviously cuts out all the packaging and all the food miles. In a subtle way, it also gives you a closer sense of understanding of the plants you are growing – especially if you are not killing the plant in harvesting from it, as the radish example indicates, where harvesting the young pods and allowing some pods to self-seed produces a much greater crop than if one harvests the root.

The importance of wild foods is that they've had no nurturing so they are strong and healthy as they are, where they are. They are native food plants. By eating them you are building that vital, vibrant, wild energy and strength into your body.

See *Food For Free*, Richard Mabey, or *Wild Food*, by Roger Phillips (Appendix 3).

Growing Foods to Cook

I am not including much on this topic because there are plenty of excellent permaculture books that will help you with both the growing techniques and types of plants to grow if you want to cook them (e.g. *Plants for a Future*, by Ken Fern, and Patrick Whitefield's books). What I will say however is that, as with nutrition, it is far healthier, easier and more multi-functional to grow starchy tubers and roots than grains. It is far easier and better for the soil to grow foods that you can cook very simply (i.e. just cleaning them and then cooking them unprocessed with their skins, such as potatoes) than to even consider growing your own grains to make some kind of bread or pasta (which when you actually think about it involves a huge amount of processing, energy, additional ingredients, baking equipment and infrastructure, etc).

Squashes and many other starchy vegetables can be eaten raw or cooked. Chilacoyote is a crazy (as in fun) plant to grow – very productive, and stores for years – that can be baked, boiled or steamed (you'll need space for it though). Even with a small garden, on a hygienist type diet (i.e. without meat, grains or dairy) of 70% raw or more, you can achieve extremely high levels of self-reliance in your food production, even in northern climates,

---

[61] Nettles are hugely nutritious and can be eaten raw by carefully picking the top few leaves, with finger and thumb on the underside at the base of the leaves; then folding the leaves together and rolling them carefully between finger and thumb... delicious, and a great picnic/party trick!

growing root vegetables in an intensive and diverse multi-layered forest garden/permaculture system. This will have fantastic ripple effects. And if you find you are eating more raw by the time your root harvest comes around you can always trade your potatoes (or whatever) for some fruits or salads, or give them away as gifts, encouraging friends and family to cut out the grains!

The *Forest Gardening* video supplied by Permanent Publications provides a wealth of inspiration on growing foods to eat both raw and cooked, with Michael and Julia Guerra being a fantastic example of the productivity that can be achieved quite easily with just a small garden. If you want a video I recommend this one highly, as it also features Robert Hart and Ken Fern, and includes a great deal of useful information on plants and the design of forest garden systems. Two other excellent videos are *The Global Gardener* and *In Grave Danger of Falling Food*, both featuring Bill Mollison.

If you are really being serious about stopping your food habits that are environmentally damaging switch to growing your own root vegetables to cook, and leave the grain products behind. If you insist on growing some grains then millet, quinoa and amaranth are good to try (and are good to sprout, which is the easiest form of grain processing); oats are a less un-natural grain for more northerly climates, and can simply be eaten rolled.

Your Permaculture Tool Bag

On a permaculture course you will develop a metaphorical 'Permaculture Tool Bag', which is a whole bunch of tools and techniques that you can use to help design your life, your house and your garden or growing space to be more sustainable and more naturally healthy. Already by reading this far in the book you have gained a very basic knowledge of your first tools in your permaculture tool bag:

* The permaculture ethics and principles.

* Zones, sectors and slope.

* Mulched beds, and soil improving plants.

* Perennials and self-seeders.

* Pick-n-pluck and cut-n-come-again salads.

* The forest garden, and staking in time and space: canopy, under-storey, shrubs and bushes, the herbaceous layer, ground cover plants, climbers and root crops.

* Companion planting and guilds.

* OBREDIM, and the design process.

When you start to think about using these tools together you may start to get some sense of how useful they can be. You can also design by looking at particular themes, such as plants, water, energy, structures or even events. You can use visualisation techniques and visioning to imagine what your established permaculture system might look like ten years in the future. You can consider the inputs and the outputs of the key elements in your design, and then make as much use as possible by developing the connections between those elements, making sure each output becomes an input for another element (i.e. kitchen scraps and garden waste goes to the compost heap or to create mulch, and the compost or mulch feeds the soil, which feeds the veg and fruit plants, which feed the people, whose 'humanure' can be composted to feed the garden, and so on.) You can also design by considering and planning how to remove the factors that are limiting your productivity in the garden, your productivity in general in life, or that are limiting your health. You can then act to remove or significantly reduce those factors, and replace them with things that increase productivity and health.

So there are in fact many approaches to design and design tools that can be used, and the best way to find out about them is to do a permaculture course. *Introduction to Permaculture* (Bill Mollison, Tagari Press) is probably the best book for getting a feel for these things. Going on a course is even better and the best possible thing you can do for understanding how the various design methods and tools work in practice.

You can consult permaculture magazines and websites to find the exciting range of permaculture courses now on offer. If you find you really enjoy it, you can even go on to do a 2 year permaculture diploma.

NASTURTIUM

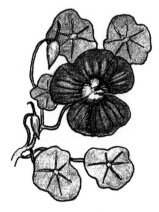

Part Three:
There Is Plenty of Information and Inspiration Out There

This section of the book includes some contributions from particularly inspiring and wise friends, and from those that are just getting on and doing it! In particular, this section is dedicated to Robert Hart, who died in 2000, age 86. In effect Robert 'invented' the concept of the forest garden; this being recognised with an award from the Institute for Social Inventions. He lived simply for many years, developing the most complete and well established forest garden in Britain at his home in Shropshire. Robert inspired, encouraged and informed literally thousands of people who came to visit his garden and who read his many books and articles. He also encouraged me very strongly to write this book.

The Forest Garden Diet
By Robert A de J Hart

When I first took over my small organic farm on Wenlock Edge in Shropshire I had two main enterprises:

1. Rearing dairy heifers for sale after calving.

2. The provision of nourishing food for my invalid mother, brother and myself.

Over the years I have learnt a great deal, by study and experience, about farming, gardening, human health and nutrition.

The ideal diet for positive health, I am convinced, consists mainly of fresh or sun-dried fruit, vegetables and herbs, consumed 70% raw. Fruit sugars feed the brain and energise the body, while chlorophyll, the green pigment which has a chemical constitution similar to that of human blood, uses solar radiation to create carbohydrates and this is the basis of physical life.

In striving to develop a system of land-working which could supply the core ingredients of such a diet throughout the year, in restricted areas and with minimum labour, I have discovered that the time-honoured system known as forest gardening or home gardening, which is practised in many countries, is the most effective, imitating, as it does, the natural forest.

One of the basic dishes of the forest garden at Highwood Hill is the 'sallet', comprising a wide variety of fruit, vegetables, nuts and herbs, as consumed in the Great Age of Herbalism, in the 17th century. As the palate gets accustomed to the strong, vital flavours of raw plant foods, the more delicious and satisfying they become.

One ceases to crave for animal foods and cereals, which undoubtedly have a clogging and acidifying effect on the system and therefore, sooner or later, lead to degenerative disease. The 'fruit and greenery' diet is alkaline and eliminative and therefore maintains the free and sweet circulation of the blood and other bodily fluids, which is an outstanding feature of positive health.

From painful experience, I learned that the provision of dairy products involves as much cruelty and slaughter as the provision of meat. In particular, the separation of the newborn calf from its mother, which is essential for milk-production, is a traumatic experience for both cow and calf. Out of compassion, as well as for health reasons, I have been a vegan for some 15 years.

I also avoid gluten cereals – wheat, barley, oats, and rye – as the protein, gluten, undoubtedly has a clogging effect on the blood-stream, leading to a build-up of toxins. Favouring, as I do, minimum cooking, I avoid baked and fried foods; the only cooking I do is to lightly boil roots and certain other vegetables in spring water, which I thicken with maize flour, millet or gram (ground lentils).

The forest garden diet is part of a compassionate, non-consumerist and sustainable lifestyle, which involves conservation of the environment and involves a sense of close communion with nature. If it were generally adopted, disease and malnutrition throughout the world could be reduced to a minimum.

If forest gardening and agroforestry become much more widespread, both in 'developed' and 'developing' nations, then the 'bioregions', which are the life-supporting areas surrounding residential centres, can be developed in such a way as to ensure regular supplies of fresh plant foods, timbers, fibres and other useful materials for everyone – town dwellers and countryfolk alike. This can be the basis on which a diverse, sophisticated, bountiful, beautiful, sustainable and positively healthy 21st century cultures can thrive.

Robert Hart, 1913-2000.

Free and Natural Life: On the Trail of Simplicity and Love
By Sibila (translated from Spanish by Steve Charter)

Listening to Instinct
To bring myself closer and closer to oneness with the Whole – this is my one search. I know I have felt this oneness in small sparks of light in my life: *I am ONE with the WHOLE, the Universe is in me and I in it because we are the same...* My desire is to live in this feeling not temporarily but with constant conscience, constant fullness... And as I know clearly that I am the whole, the way that turns out to be most direct to obtain my goal is to connect with *me*, with my essence.

As a result, to allow myself to be me, I arrive at emptiness, the one thing that immediately fills the whole... To be faithful to this path I cannot have an existence based in external things, other people, books, and so on. They serve me sometimes as ideas to consider and as a way to explore my own experience, until I am able to see if their truth runs through my veins; if I feel its truth in a way that leads me to want to welcome it into my life. Other people can help me to understand and appreciate some things better, although I do not necessarily need to be drawn to do as they do.

Initially, this way of being flowed in me from within; without me being conscious of it, without me questioning my inability to follow idols, gurus or teachers, whether in music, visual arts, literature, in nutrition, clothes or spirituality. I liked to read everything and from everything I gained and welcomed something but nothing in particular married me to one path. This attitude together with a strong feeling for solitude alongside my lack of self-understanding and my lack of knowing how to feel and to live life, as much in family surroundings as in the society in which we lived, took me more and more to what my parents called 'living in a turtle's shell'.

From adolescence, my best friend was always a newspaper which questioned everything and that helped me to investigate more and more my feelings, to explore them in their deepest sense. And so I began to listen to my instinct and little by little everything was changing drastically in me.

Already I was valueing things differently, to avoid suffering in vain, and I came to learn the lesson of detachment. Detachment towards the family, friends, sex, possessions... and even food and the culture in which I lived. When you go more and more intimately within yourself, relying on yourself more and more and, therefore connect more to Nature (and therefore yourself), your life becomes simpler little by little. Within that simplicity for me there is no place for cooking food and everything that it entails.

If I now think about buying food and detergent, the conventional cleaning of a conventional house, cooking, mopping, preparing the table, feeding the children at set times, and so on, it's very clear. Heavens! What a pile of work! And all this to soil my body and mind as well as to cloud my energy. Rarely have I eaten something cooked in the last two years. When I have (and in two cases with animal products – namely cheese on pizzas), I have quickly felt a much more dense energy and have felt less harmonious or fluid with the Universe. I no longer felt fully responsible in my actions, instead I felt a soiling of my blood and, therefore, my brain and heart.

When I truly see clearly and feel the energy of things, I discover that when I eat something the energy and the feelings of it fuses with me. If I eat something with a very low vibration like something cooked, my body requires concerted efforts to turn it into life, a higher vibration, draining me of certain minerals and using a great deal of vital energy to process that food.

Then, I listen to my body that says to me, that shouts to me: I want simplicity!

I believe that there are many ways and/or reasons to arrive at eating raw foods. You can arrive after reading and taking in a good theoretical book, or you can arrive from a desperate search to recover lost health after many diverse but unsuccesful attempts at other ways of living. Or you can arrive through a cast-iron desire not to consume anything that entails materialism (economy, work dependency, state finance and control, environmental contamination, consumer distractions...). Or simply you can listen to your instinct.

Taking myself to live in nature without a house with heating, was a decisive act for me. I connected so much with myself that simplicity just appeared and the chains were broken. Then, quite simply there was already no place for cooking. My previous life began to be incongruous to me on many levels – for example, taking part in diverse activities to stop global warming but, at the same time contributing still more to it whenever I cooked – realising by this time that this is only a habit, and that in addition that it is harmful.

The more I removed myself the more centered I have been and the more connected to Nature, the less I needed anything cooked. Here, in my home, in the countryside, the choice is easy: Why contaminate, or damage the body, fill myself with junk and things like casseroles, to create things to clean (pans, plates, cutlery, body and mind!), to increase stress and to waste time cooking, buying and cleaning when my children and I can go to one pear tree and eat when we desire and the amount that we want? That really is clean, comfortable, simplicity and freedom! There is always something throughout year that can be picked ripe or stored, and if we buy something it is with conscience and knowing full well that fruit – if it has been stored, is fresh off the tree or it is wild – has been made by nature to be beneficial to us.

If you begin to listen and to allow yourself to be yourself, the fullness of life will invade your being. Although in the beginning you may feel some tears for people, customs or things that will disappear from your life, that is only temporary. It will be fully replaced by an eternal fullness born of simplicity and freedom, a love of life and the non-living things – a love of the connection with Nature and the Universe, with yourself and with the Whole... Then raw eating, life in the countryside, nudism, simplicity, organic living, the extended family, heightened senses and many other things will little by little come one-by-one, without pain, making clear to you that all these aspects comprise just one single law – the Law of Universal Energy and Love.

For me raw food is not only a question of health, it is much more than that. It is a powerful questioning, and is a spiritual path as well as one that brings a more simple life, that frees my essence, in search of my original self. The path of that search is one of sincerity and purity, allowing me to be myself, through instinct. Listening to my instinct I am following my own path. I am my own guru and teacher. She or he is really wise who only obeys universal laws faithfully and thereby benefits from them. And, if sometimes I do not follow them, it is not from ignorance of that law, but by being conscious of my emotional and psychic limitations, that are not instinctive. In these cases, I choose to feed the ego or my dependencies without forgetting or letting myself have the light radiated by my instinct present, by my inner wisdom that, with its single presence allows me to be less chained in my life every day.

Looking For Simplicity

By following this path, I went to live in the countryside, I chose nakedness whereever possible, to sleep outside, to eat raw, not to have a car, telephone or any rubbish, and so on. By doing so, little by little, I found I was connecting more and more with myself, with my own innate light and wisdom, with joy and fullness breaking through in my life. Optimism, universal love and heightened senses flooded my being... No longer did I have depressions, bad moods and dark thoughts or feelings – I found instead a deep pool of light and love, of fullness, wisdom and healing, and of optimism.

The more we connect with our interior, the more we connect to it still. This is the the way I arrived at raw eating. I had not only not read a single book on the subject, but neither did I know of the concept of the 'raw fooder', or of other people who eat this way, and of the physiological benefits of doing so. In other words, I did not know of the theoretical basis that suggests that humans are naturally frugivorous, not omnivorous. Discovering all this arrived later and was a surprise for me. How fascinating it turns out to be to discover one day your true family, your spiritual family...! My heart almost exploded with the connection I felt!

I talk of the people who eat raw and, in particular, of raw vegans, as my spiritual family not just because of the food they eat, but also of the other things that eating this way entails. I see also a side effect of this more natural way of eating that involves a way of feeling and understanding so specific to life that it does not accept another alternative. It is a way of feeling, an understanding of life and a philosophy of life that led me to eat this way.

My love towards animals and being conscious of the fear and the suffering experienced by all those that are going to be eaten, led me not to want to eat them. If I did not eat animals, less of them would be sacrificed. I had fears, many of them, about my physical health because of the cultural pressure that often has a powerful presence within an adolescent, as I was at that time. But whenever I ate animals, my soul cried bitterly and painfully. I was determined. Now I only had to break my psychic and emotional dependencies. I trusted in the passage of time for this, as well as in the sincerity of the feelings of my heart. Later, after more and more feelings of connection with Nature and all its beings, I felt that I began to communicate once in a while with the plants – I also began to question the necessity of their sacrifice for my survival and began to believe in the possibilities of devine Pranic nutrition. Again, I had to allow more time and to trust myself.

Eating vegetarian, little by little I was questioning the global warming by our daily acts like smoking cigarettes or joints (which I did not do), driving and cooking (which I did) and began to wish not to contribute to it any more. My instinct was calling for more and more simplicity and, little by little, I was moving away from the complications of cooking. I had children and through all this I really enjoyed my increasing consciousness of money and energy saving as well as the freedom and comfort that came from not cooking.

Now I have the memory of that daily life in which I worked seven hours away from home, I studied at university, I had an infinity of diverse possessions and clothes that required a lot of work to look after (work for money and the physical work of looking after things), as well as cleaning. Almost every day I had dedicated between two and four hours to the kitchen, making elaborate and diverse dishes, making bread, yogurt, cheese, seitán, tofu, cakes and other complicated things. Dedicating as much routine time to all those things, I ask myself now where was there space left for me - and thank heavens I did not have a television! Now I see that at that time my life was very poor spiritually, too materialistic and superficial. Yes, I enjoyed doing all those things and some of those possessions but now, with the passage of the years, I have seen that they offer diversion but not a fullness in life, because they *are* diversions, born of a culture, not of the heart, the instinct or nature... They are diversions that are great chains to our being and, although we learn to live with them, they do not stop being chains. Definitely, I prefer freedom and freedom always comes with simplicity.

When I find a doubt about whether I did something by instinct or culture, I ask myself how I would have acted in such a case 25, 30 or 50 centuries passed... and, then, always I see the light. As a result of this light, I decide, and I decide with conscience, not by inertia. If I choose by how I would have acted centuries before, I see no advantages in the decisions and things that I was tied to before – and in this way I have decided not to do those things anymore. If I choose according to the standard cultural guidelines, then I find I am not being responsible for my actions, including my unhealthy dependencies and blockages, as well as my habits. In these situations I remind myself that I am capable of everything – I only have to know clearly what I want, to give time for this to happen and to trust. To trust Love and Universal Energy, to trust myself.

Sibila (Nuria Aragon Castro)

The above is from the introduction to Sibila's first book: *Vida Libre y Natural: en el sendero de la sencillez y el amor* (Free and Natural Life: on the trail of simplicity and love). See Appendix 3.

Indoor Gardening and Living Foods

This section is compiled from an article by Elaine Bruce in *Permaculture Magazine* No.9, and an interview with Elaine in *The FRESH Network News*, Feb - April, 1999.

The wonderful benefits of indoor gardening should not be ignored when considering both raw food nutrition and permaculture. We can use window sills and shelves, and all sorts of indoor spaces, to grow many plants. Indoor gardening is an important part of a 'Living Foods Lifestyle' that aims for 'super nutrition' by supplying fresh organic foods, with the extra dimension of enzyme rich and chlorophyll rich foods. This is a very powerful way of helping the body's own enzymes in repairing cells and boosting immunity.

To supply these powerful healing and cleansing foods with relatively little effort in particular involves growing both quantities of sprouted seeds (e.g. alfalfa, green lentils, mung beans, chick peas, radish, quinoa, etc.) and good amounts of 'indoor greens' (young shoots, such as sunflower, radish or buckwheat) which can be eaten in salads, in cold green energy soups or juiced.

Sprouting in jars and trays is a relatively easy way to supply a large quantity of these top quality foods, all organic, and at a low cost – especially if you buy in bulk, perhaps with friends, from a wholefood co-op. All you have to do with most seeds is soak them over-night and rinse them daily. Depending on the temperature and type, your delicious sprouts will be ready in two, three or four days – voila! Green lentils, chick peas and quinoa are quick sprouters; mung beans and alfalfa take a day or so more.

Chlorophyll, which is concentrated in the leaves of 'indoor greens' and wheat grass in particular, is especially powerful in detoxifying the body and rebuilding living tissue. This is probably because its chemical structure is almost identical to that of haemoglobin in blood. Wheat-grass juice (i.e. the green juice from sprouted wheat grain shoots, grown in a tray on a thin bed of compost) is the ultimate chlorophyll provider. The powerful green juice is squeezed out of the grass using special manual or electric juicers.[62]

Dr. Ann Wigmore, who established the Living Foods Programme, was a lively, dynamic person. Shining with health and vitality, she was totally focused on her teaching. She always went straight to the root of the problem. She expected staff to be efficient without fuss in the running of the gardens, planting sheds, marketing, catering and basic classes. With her guests she was equally straightforward. She assumed they were prepared to work hard to regain their health, always encouraging them to take their green drinks and to have faith in their own ability to heal. She also believed in the power of love to heal, and this showed in her manner of answering questions. She would not collude with people who tried to get her approval to cut corners!

Ann Wigmore and her associates have taught many people around the world. So the normal route to living foods is via a course, perhaps inspired by one of the many inspiring books on the subject. Living foods courses are an enjoyable blend of practical hands-on sessions and theory. They start with the basics of growing a complete range of sprouted seeds and year-round indoor greens – good use of Zone 0 (i.e. inside the house) in permaculture terms.

Many recipes and techniques are demonstrated on a course in order to give all the information needed to establish a Living Foods kitchen. The processes of fermentation and dehydration are explained and freshly made dishes are served immediately with an abundance of fresh organic produce. Emphasis is placed on the uses of chlorophyll as the most efficient and inexpensive way to maintain health and vitality. The courses also look at detoxification and

---

[62] Steve's note: It is even possible to combine the Living Foods and 'Food For Free' concepts by using the lawn or a patch of nettles as a green juice factory!

healing, and how to manage the transition process to Living Foods.

The Living Foods perspective is generally sympathetic to the ideal of fruit-arianism, with some doubts about it's appropriateness in a temperate climate for large numbers of people. Elaine's personal experience is of unbounded energy, disease resistance and stress tolerance on lots of raw green foods and drinks. Thousands of people have reversed serious ill health and life threatening problems and regained normal health and strength on the Living Foods Programme.

Elaine would not normally advise fasting, believing it's unnecessary on the Living Foods Programme. Fasting is a natural and instinctive thing to do in acute illness and fever, but prolonged fasting, or fasting undertaken for other reasons, should only be done after an objective assessment from an experienced and sympathetic practitioner who can give individual advice. In working with nature it is critical to understand that the body is programmed to self-heal, and to survive. It sets its own priorities, and when suddenly tipped into deep cleansing, the end results may not be as expected.

A Living Foods kitchen with its indoor garden takes no more daily time than cooker or freezer based routines; more time is spent on washing salads and scrubbing veggies and on daily care of indoor greens and sprouts. This is more than offset by time saved on shopping, storage, preparing/cooking and washing up.

Wheatgrass has a very important role in a living foods diet. Wholefood stores sell a wide range of wheatgrass supplements, but these are processed and therefore not at all natural.

Wheatgrass juice has to be taken freshly pressed, within 20 minutes. Powdered, freeze-dried products cannot possibly achieve the amazing reversal of disease processes that fresh chlorophyll, in conjunction with the rest of the Living Foods Programme, can. They are at most an emergency food supplement when travelling, but are emphatically not a substitute for the fresh juice.

In Elaine's Living Foods kitchen you will find...

INDOOR GREENS grown in trays of compost. The seeds of sunflower and buckwheat are most popular, although radish and even fenugreek can be used. These are soaked, allowed to germinate, and then spread to grow on the surface of compost laid thinly on a tray. They are kept in the dark (damp but not wet) for a few days and then put in the window racks to green for a few days. They are then ready to be cut near the base to be eaten fresh and vital in salads or juiced in green drinks. Indoor greens provide cheap, excellent quality fresh organic greens, full of natural nutrients, throughout the year.

WHEATGRASS is grown in the same way. After some days when it has grown to perhaps six inches, it is cut and juiced to give a daily dose of healthy vitamins, especially the anti-oxidants, and plant enzymes. Fresh chlorophyll both nourishes and cleanses the tissues and helps to protect against radiation and chemical pollution. Hand powered wheatgrass juicers are very affordable for those that want to avoid electrical equipment.

SPROUTED SEEDS are kept in jars, with plenty of room for air and growth. It is best to use a wide range. This can include crunchy sprouts like chickpeas and lentils, soft sweet ones like aduki and mung, hot or spicy ones like mustard and fenugreek, and the best one of all for vitamins – alfalfa. Sprouted seeds and nuts are used both as they are and in recipes for raw patés, humous, tabbouleh, seed loaves and nut cheese. Some are made into dehydrator crisps and cookies, both sweet and savoury – these are particularly good for those in transition to a raw living foods diet.

SURPLUS PRODUCE from the garden can be dehydrated and stored. Sliced dried tomatoes and onions make wonderful flavourings. Raspberries, sliced peaches, apricots, and wild blackberries can be reconstituted in a little spring water for fruit salads in winter.

JUICERS are used daily to make green drinks and vegetable and fruit juices.

FERMENTED FOODS are also an important item: sauerkraut, rejuvelac (fermented wheat grain soaked in water), and seed cheeses.

A few things are very gently cooked. Millet, sometimes known as 'the Queen of grains' is a seed used as an alkalinising grain substitute, and is very useful for those in transition. It only needs a short spell of low heat to soften the seed coats. Sometimes a potassium broth is used to regulate the acid/alkaline balance of the body.

A Green Drink for Winter

Juice one part celery to two parts spinach or leaf beet, plus a carrot or beetroot/beet for added richness and taste. Or, for a lighter drink, add half an apple instead of the carrot/beet or beetroot.

Elaine Bruce has been practising and teaching the Living Foods Programme for many years. She was originally taught by Dr. Ann Wigmore, in Boston in 1980, and joined her staff at the Puerto Rico Clinic for a time in 1992. She has trained and studied intensively in Naturopathy and Homeopathy. Currently, Elaine runs courses from her home in Shropshire on how to set up a Living Foods kitchen, and the complete Living Foods lifestyle. Elaine herself has been on a Living Foods diet for eighteen years, and 100% raw for most of that time. She is also a trained permaculture designer, with a very neat and efficient urban permaculture garden – indoors and out.

Specialist books on Living Foods and sprouting, as well as wheatgrass juicers and other juicers are available from Elaine or the FRESH Network – see Appendix 3.

Paradise Gardening

The following has been distilled from a slightly longer article by Joe Hollis

Paradise is, first of all, a garden – one in which everything we need is there for the taking. Paradise Gardening is a way of life which maintains the garden, and which in turn is maintained by that garden; a way of living that uses a small fraction of the available energy, whilst serving the functioning and continued survival of the garden ecosystem.

Paradise Gardening is not work, in the same way that what a bear does during the day is 'not work'. Paradise Gardening is not agriculture – it is a habitat and a niche; our place, our fit. How does a bird build its nest? With so many factors to consider it just picks the most beautiful spot. Like any other creature, we are our niche. By our physiology and behaviour we are born to live a certain kind of life. Paradise garden is a way both to deliver our birthright and within which to fulfil our duty.

Everything needed to be completely human is available to us in the environment – the garden and the neighbourhood. We can rely on this because 'human-ness' is a creation of the environment. You and I are recent manifestations of a co-evolution between our genes and all the other genes 'out there' – a co-evolution that began with the start of life on earth.

When we live in Paradise Garden we are specialists of working with nature to help create and sustain diversity. This type of foraging lifestyle is now widely recognised as a superior adaptation to agriculture – a revolution in the study of the human niche emerged from the realisation that foragers, far from living on the brink of starvation, actually have more leisure than anyone else. Agriculture has increased production, but only at the cost of even greater increases in labour and other inputs, such as energy and agro-chemicals. Other costs also come from reduced dietary quality (because of loss of diversity), and greater risk of losing the harvest to pests or bad weather.

In the modern world clearly there can be no going back to foraging. However, there can be going forward to Paradise Gardening – which can be described as 'intensified foraging'. This is a move from massive agricultural manipulation of ecosystems, to more subtle transformation of ecosystems. This involves the alteration of selected components of the natural system rather than its wholesale replacement. It is a method of cultivation which places certain preferred species in particularly suitable ecological niches, to simulate the structures and dynamics of the natural ecosystem. This is based on the realisation that "many 'non-agricultural' people were in fact engaged in intensive and sophisticated plant exploitation, previously unrecognised because their plant management practices did not fit into our idea of agriculture." (Harris, Ed. *From Foraging To Farming*)

On this path, our goal is to 'naturalise' ourselves in the environment, by changing ourselves and the environment to an ecological 'fit' that suits both. Perfect fit means a free and easy flow of matter and energy – life lived as a complete and balanced gift, from the garden to us, and from us to the garden.

What we need *now* is a process that leads us to that garden; a process that is justified in its own terms. Seeking the 'ideal' Paradise Garden will only perpetuate the same old patterns of selling out the present for some imagined better future. Ecology and permaculture teach that a pioneer (disturbed) environment favours the fast-growing but short-lived plants, those designed to capture the most light and unoccupied soil – wide spreading and 'greedy'. Eventually they are replaced by trees, which are more stable, longer lived and finally faster growing, more influential and the dominant species. We are widespread and greedy; evolution and natural succession indicate that eventually the 'competitive advantage' will pass to those that practise permanence, rootedness, slow growth and steady accumulation, with vertical expansion of the human spirit into uncharted or long-forgotten realms.

Paradise Gardening involves extricating our life-support systems from 'civilisation'/the economy (bluntly money) and re-attaching it to the natural world of the garden and the neighbourhood. This is a gradual process requiring a deep analysis of our needs and expenditures (of physical, emotional and mental energy, as well as of money). So cars and petrol are no longer seen as needs, but only as means to satisfy needs – means which can be changed relatively easily. The solution, for example, is to reduce the need to travel (which is usually to get or spend money).

The Tao Te Ching says:
'The country over the border may be so close that one could hear the cocks crowing and the dogs barking in it, but the people would grow old and die without ever once troubling to go there.'

Whilst things made by the 'system' may be technically superior, things made by one's own efforts will have a superior quality that can be called 'heart'. Satisfaction of needs by the system normally declines rapidly after the moment of purchase. Needs met through our own interaction with nature are more deeply met, with wonderful surprises along the way – as most people that have made anything 'from scratch' will know. What seldom occurs to us is that an entire life can be lived in this way; through a re-integration of needs. Food, exercise, healing, entertainment, learning, creativity, spiritual inspiration – all these needs can be met by the garden at the same time.

Enriching the garden by naturalising useful and beautiful species and learning to incorporate them into our lives begins, of course, with the present and potential 'natural' vegetation. To this are added species from similar ecosystems worldwide, with slight habitat enhancements. This brings about possibilities for new species; a 'cornucopia' never available to previous generations. 'Planned biotic enrichment' is within our power – to not only hold down the rate of species extinction but to reverse it, through 'species packing' that creates assorted equilibria that exceed any occurring in nature. This game of life involves creating new (biotic) communities and ecosystem transformations that offer creative work with huge benefits to people, place and planet.

We live within a narrow 'window of opportunity' – and we cannot put off our choice for any more lifetimes. A revolutionary shift in consciousness and lifestyle is needed. We have little time to achieve this transition – before long the environment will be too degraded, the soils too depleted, the waters too polluted, the resources lost, with too many species extinct, and a human population that has increased massively. Within this context the paper tiger of more trade and economic growth just cannot deliver.

We all have two hands, one lifetime, twenty-four hours a day. This democratic factor means that working by hand on a small piece of land (which could be local 'public' land), we can create a Paradise with relevance for all. Paradise Gardening is vastly more meaningful than any bio-dome experiment to a world in need of examples that show a 'better' way – a sustainable, democratic and life-enhancing way.

For a section on local practice and details of a newsletter contact:

Joe Hollis, Mountain Gardens, 3020 White Oak Creek Road, Burnsville, NC 28714. USA. Joe Hollis also co-ordinates the Permaculture Seed and Plant Exchange. For more information on his personal approach to paradise gardening, permaculture and seed saving you can visit Joe Hollis' excellent webpage at http://webpages.charter.net/czar207196/garden.htm

Plants for a Future

A knowledge of the Plants For A Future concept and the project is highly relevant in linking raw food nutrition with permaculture. The concept is that we can, with knowledge, meet all of our needs from plants and plant products – and if we do so much more than we are now, it will be a very positive move for people and planet.

Plants for a Future (PFAF) is a non-profit making charitable education and research project, and a workers co-operative. The project supplies information on useful perennial plants that can be grown in a temperate climate. Where possible the project also aims to supply these plants through the workers co-operative. All the plants are grown without the use of artificial fertilisers, sprays or animal products. PFAF is a registered charity (Charity Number 1057719).

PFAF was established in 1989 at Penpol near Lostwithiel in Cornwall to grow and demonstrate the wide range of useful plants that can be grown outdoors in Britain. This followed years of research into plant uses – both information gathering and the collecting and growing of plants themselves. They now have around 1,700 varieties of edible and otherwise useful plants growing at 'the Field'. It was a degraded empty barley field when they bought it. Now it is a deep, lush food forest which also provides many other needs such as wood, fibres and soap plants. PFAF have compiled a database of around 7000 such species. The database, catalogue and information sheets are all available to the public, and many of their plants are supplied by mail order. The project has an excellent website, which includes the database.

PFAF now have an additional 80 acre (36 hectare) site in north Devon and have established a research and education centre. Having secured planning permission for their demonstration gardens and a research centre in 2000, PFAF intends to become a model for the diversification of rural land-use through the development of a sustainable and integrated economic, educational and ecological project – a place for both living and working in harmony with the rural environment.

PFAF also have a plant advisory service, which can be based on a visit by Ken Fern (author of the excellent book *Plants For A Future*, Permanent Publications), or a postal advice service. For certain demonstration or research projects PFAF may supply plants on a cost only basis, and design advice – anyone interested in becoming a demonstration garden or a regional research site should contact PFAF.

The PFAF education and research charity has the following aims and objectives. Please give Plants For A Future your support, as they really deserve it. Do what you can to help seed and spread the PFAF concept all around the world to every climate zone!

PFAF Aims and Objectives (Summarised)

✳ To advance the education of the public by promoting all aspects of ecologically sustainable, vegan-organic horticulture and agriculture with an emphasis on tree, shrub and other perennial species; with research into such agriculture and horticulture undertaken by the workers co-operative, and the promotion and dissemination of the results research by the educational charity.

✳ PFAF's land aims to provide a home to a wide variety of creatures that are unable to obtain all their food, security and shelter needs from conventional agriculture.

For more information contact: PFAF Research & Visitor Centre, Blagdon Cross, near Holsworthy, Devon. See: http://www.scs.leeds.ac.uk/pfaf/ Tel: 01409 211694 or 01208 873554.

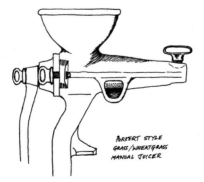

PORKERT STYLE
GRASS/WHEATGRASS
MANUAL JUICER

The Conclusion:
This Is The Beginning Not The End...

Dietary choice and your overall lifestyle need good information, a good deal of thought, and some careful and extended observation. At times it may also be good for you to let go of your thoughts and just try listening to your body; to sense what feels natural and 'right'.

For me this has meant looking at information on raw/living foods, alongside other dietary information, and information on food growing and my lifestyle in general; as well as trusting my body's 'innate intelligence' to tell me what feels good. There is no question that it works. So I use my mind and my body to get a feel for where I am now (in a lifestyle and philosophical sense), and where I am going. I then identify and follow the practical next steps that feel right for me.

If you choose to explore the 'Working With Nature' path the FRESH[63] (Fruitarian and Raw Energy Support and Help) Network, Living Nutrition/ Healthy Living International and Nature's First Law on the raw side, and The Permaculture Association (UK) or many of the US permaculture organisations on the sustainable lifestyles side can assist significantly. FRESH, for example, was established for People Care reasons – to provide good information, based on personal experience and detailed research, and to provide support and networking for those exploring a high proportion of raw food or fruitarian diet. This is achieved through an excellent magazine, a superb website, lively e-groups, a mail order book list which supplies a fantastic variety of books, many of which are imported and otherwise difficult to find in the UK, and through various gatherings, lectures, courses and local groups. I certainly hope that a lot of wisdom can be shared between the permaculture community and the natural diet/raw food community. At least once a year the nearest raw food and permaculture groups in an area, town or city, should have a combined gathering, have fun, and learn from each other.

For permaculture information and support there are a great range of groups that cover all regions of the USA, and the Permaculture Association in the UK, which now has an extensive network of local groups, and many activities linked with permaculture courses and education, an Associated Projects network and a whole range of other supportive activities including a newsletter *Permaculture Works*. A huge number of peoples' lives have been changed very positively by discovering permaculture – in Britain and Europe, in Australia where it started, in the USA, and now increasingly in many of the economically poorer countries around the world, with some great and inspiring projects in Nepal, India, Africa and South America.

Permanent Publications is a publishing company and is separate from the

---

[63] The FRESH Network: contact details inside back cover, web site: www.eclipse.co.uk/fresh

Association, but a very close friend! They produce a quarterly *Permaculture Magazine* which is a superb source of information, and they publish an excellent range of books on permaculture, sustainability and simple living. They also produce the *Earth Repair Catalogue* which is a fantastically useful mail order book service that covers a vast range of relevant and inter-related subjects. Both the Association and the Magazine have excellent websites of course, with a large selection of useful and inspiring permaculture links. Chelsea Green in the USA produce and sell a similarly excellent range of sustainable living books, and *The Permaculture Activist* magazine is a great starting place to find your way into the north American permaculture world.

Thanks to such organisations, and despite what I thought more than nine years ago now, I now know that I can survive, and even thrive and be healthier and happier, on a high percentage raw foods diet – AND, I can grow a lot more of my own food than I would have thought possible years ago, organically and at very low cost. Personally, I have been amazed how well permaculture ethics and principles apply to diet and my lifestyle as a whole. I'm only starting to glimpse the implications of permaculture design and working with nature in Zone oo – looking at my 'whole nutrition', what I feed my mind, body, emotions and spirit, and how far I can go in designing that to be positive and naturally healthy!

Either consciously or unconsciously, we all do a lot of designing of our own lifestyles – image, work and career, home and garden, mode of transport, pastimes and of course the food we eat. So I humbly suggest that in designing your own lifestyle you base your food and dietary choices on a good variety of quality information, and on careful observation through actual experience. This may mean challenging your preconceptions and looking into a high percentage organic raw food diet, alongside other dietary information. Cut out TV and newspapers for example and replace them with positive, healthy and creative nutrition for your mind, spirit and emotions – such as appropriate books, magazines, videos, CDs and tapes, networks and friends.

My choices about what I eat have certainly changed since I was given what, from my own experience and observation, I consider to be good, non-dogmatic and non-extremist, positive, rational information about what I now see as a more natural and positive way of life. In fact it has blown several of my 'reality tunnels' to pieces – a positive experience that has helped me to see some of my other blocks to learning. And I just feel so much better for it, in so many ways. Above all it feels like it is working with nature.

Shift From Consuming Life to Producing Abundance

If you link forest gardening with the Plants For A Future[64] concept, permaculture thinking, indoor gardening, intuitive eating and an understanding of raw food nutrition, with a dose of Food For Free thrown in too, it will provide you with

---

[64] See Ken Fern's book *Plants For A Future*, Permanent Publications, 1997.

the tools to take the first steps towards creating a new and liberated, vibrant and vital, health creating, sustainable and life-enhancing culture.

Change what you buy and how you use your money. Buy food and products that support moves towards greater health, in your self and in the ecological health of the planet. As much as you can, spend and invest only in ways which create greater health and sustainability. Buy foods with minimum packaging, and cut out tinned foods and other over packaged foods. Buy larger quantities of fruit and veg in boxes, and use an attractive and practical re-usable shopping bag. Buy dried seeds and pulses, and dried fruit, and again you can reduce the packaging in your waste stream. Find out about any local organic veggie box schemes that may exist, or any local organic purchasing co-operatives. And if there aren't any you could always seek out a few friends and other similarly minded people and get on with starting one yourself. Learn how to do it from others that exist happily and healthily elsewhere.

Most of all get planting. So the same goes for buying seeds, plants and trees for your garden, allotment, or for a community garden. Then you can 'Plant, Plant, Plant!' Plant in your own patch an all year vegetable, herb and salad garden; plant a forest garden – anything from a tiny mini-forest garden to a huge edible forest will do. Every little does help. Truly, every action no matter how small does have its effect, either one way or another. Choose positive, creative effects and love every minute of it – that's the paradise garden philosophy!

Plant liberally and carefully in your landscape. Co-create, diversify and expand the growing, living library of natural genetic diversity. 'Plant, Plant, Plant' to transform your patch, your neighbourhood and the whole living landscape to create a productive, healthy and sustainable global Paradise Garden! And with the will to create positive change in ourselves and the world we are part of, we can eat our way towards true health and sustainability...

Now it's over to you...

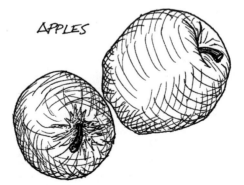

APPLES

PART FOUR:
The Appendices

Appendix 1: Some Recipes and Meal Ideas

There are many, many raw food recipe books that provide a host of wonderful dishes, both savoury and sweet, to entice the palate, to boggle the eyes and to make the taste buds dance with joy[64]. Rather than include a huge long list of recipes, I have provided some of the basics that I have found to be both really easy and really delicious.

One of the great attractions of raw eating is that once you've got the basics it is much simpler than cooking and normally involves a lot less preparation time and clearing up than cooked meals. So you don't need to know a whole bunch of complicated or special raw recipes – although you can certainly find them easily enough if that's what you're into, as 'Cordon Raw' is now very fashionable in California for example.

Just as in conventional eating, most people tend to rely on a relatively small number of standard meals that they rotate and vary. So if you get a good set of basic raw food meals then you are more than half way there. In my experience the difference with raw standards is that the flavour is always fresh, so they somehow never seem to taste quite the same and they're virtually always a delight to the taste buds. My aim here is to give you some starters – however, most of all I want you to experiment and feel confident about creating your own favourites, whilst also having some well-known standards. It's actually easy.

Personally I do not use any exact measurements or quantities as I have found it is much better to follow my own instinct on how much of what to include. This way I also get slightly different proportions of ingredients each time I make something, which means it tastes deliciously different every time. So some of the donated recipes below include measurements, and others do not.

STEVE'S RECIPE FOR SUCCESS

My recipe for success with salads is to make sure you have a good selection of salad vegetables through the week (home grown and/or bought), so that you can pick and choose each day according to what you fancy. Get used to using say 10 to 15 basic salad ingredients. You can then play around with different proportions of each, different mixtures, combinations and so on, using the additional flavours suggested below as you like. Some days you can leave out one, two or three ingredients, and on other you can leave out a whole bunch and just have a really simple mix of your favourites.

---

[64] Contact the FRESH Network by post or via their website to get an extensive book list with many fantastic ideas for meals and recipes, from the day-to-day basics to true cordon-bleu raw extravaganzas.

So here's a list of different salad ingredients you can go for:

* Cabbage (red and/or white).

* Carrots.

* Spinach.

* Tomatoes.

* Celery.

* Spanish (red) onion.

* Avocados.

* Red or Yellow peppers (do not use green peppers as they are not ripe).

* Rocket.

* Broccoli.

* Chicory.

* Cauliflower.

* Cucumber.

* Lettuce (e.g. Black Seeded Simpson's from Future Foods), Romaine, etc.

* Courgette/Zucchini.

* Beetroot/Beets.

* Wild greens picked from the garden or elsewhere.

On the side, the following can be useful for aiding transition to more raw foods: sea weed (e.g. dulse), olive oil, garlic, spices (chilli, cumin, etc.), ginger. Generally however, the simpler the better – do not get 'addicted' to these stimulating flavours and make sure you have plenty of meals without them. Add to your basic ingredients a good knife and chopping board, a grater and perhaps one or two gadgets like a hand mincer and hand seed grinder, a good and ideally beautiful bowl or plate or two that you enjoy eating from, and then you're away...!

Salad Success
Take the seeds of a wide range of perennial and self-seeding salad plants – these might be rocket, lettuces, endive, different kales, tomatoes, perennial spinach, chard, oriental salad greens such as Mitsuna or mustard greens, chicory, celery, lovage, etc. (see forest garden and permaculture sections for easily grown perennial vegetables), and add a few seeds of edible flowers such as nasturtiums, mallow and calendula. Sprinkle these lightly in appropriate parts of the garden, in large pots or in window boxes. Add water. Add more water according to climatic needs on the days following the day of sowing and then as needed during the growth of the plants.

Leave in the sun for 2 to 4 months, and then harvest and eat with some of the other fabulous recipes detailed below...

Some Really Delicious and Radically Healthy Recipes

These recipes have been donated by friends who support the working with nature philosophy and who have all travelled the road of transition. So they know how to prepare meals that taste great, whilst also helping our minds and bodies get used to eating differently. So without further ado, here's a bunch of great recipes for you to try.

DAVE KLEIN RECIPES

Here's four great, really simple recipes from Dave Klein, Editor of the excellent *Living Nutrition* magazine, which also has produced it's own recipe book (see Appendix 3 for contact details). I love these recipes because they show just how simple raw foods can be... and they also show that 'simple' in this case is also simply delicious. Dave lives in California so some of his recipes are more suitable to buying or growing foods that are suited to that climate.

Morning Glory
Ingredients:
* Several sweet oranges.
* 1 pomegranate.

Instructions: 1. Slice the oranges and pomegranate in half. 2. Using a citrus press or other citrus juicer, juice the fruits, then mix and enjoy!

Grape – Celery Cooler
Juice your favourite sweet grapes. After the grapes, juice 1 or 2 celery stalks per glass. Stir and serve. Garnish with mint leaves if desired. Optional: Cut a thin slice of fresh ginger root. Juice the ginger slice with the grapes.

Avo-buttered Corn On The Cob
Ingredients:
* Corn on the cob, freshly shucked.
* Avocado, halved and pitted.

Instructions: With the corn in one hand and the avocado in the other, smear the avocado over the corn kernels and enjoy! Best eaten barefooted!

Sesame Hors d'Oeuvres
Ingredients:
* Raw sesame tahini.
* Slicing cucumbers.

Instructions: 1. Slice the cucumbers into thin discs. Optional: peel the skins first. If the skins are waxed, peeling is mandatory. 2. Spoon a portion of the tahini on the cuke slices. Optional: place a cucumber slice on top of the tahini, making a mini sandwich.

SHAZZIE'S DETOX DELIGHTS RECIPES

Here's some recipes from Shazzie, a regular columnist for *Get Fresh*, the Fresh Network's magazine. For details of the great little book *Shazzie's Detox Delights* – which is very helpful for those wanting to really enjoy eating more healthily, has received 'rave reviews' from its readers, and which doesn't mention vegan or raw foods at all – you can check Shazzie's excellent website (see Appendix 3). Shazzie has lived in England (temperate climate) and southern Spain (Mediterranean climate) so some of her recipes are more suited to growing in a warmer climate. Many though are relevant for growing in both temperate and Mediterranean climates. Here are some recipes from Shazzie which are in the book, to get you dribbling...

Sweet Spread

Shazzie says: "I love this! I serve this on big romaine leaves, put basil leaves on top and eat it like an open sandwich" You can also try it with any other leaves you might grow in your salad garden.

* 1 avocado, peeled and stoned.

* 1 banana, peeled.

* 1 clove of garlic.

Chop the garlic and blend all the ingredients in a food processor or by hand of course.

Italian Soup

Shazzie says: "This is a very simple but really tasty soup. You can add other flavours to it for lots of variation."

* 1 avocado, peeled and stoned.

* 4 tomatoes.

* A handful of basil.

* 1/4 of a cup of cold pressed olive oil.

Blend all ingredients. If it's too thick add some freshly made tomato or cucumber juice.

Sunny Hemp Paté

* 1 cup of sprouted hemp seeds.

* 2 cups of sprouted sunflower seeds.

* 1 onion.

* 1 clove of garlic.

* 1 teaspoon of paprika.

* 1 teaspoon of dried mixed herbs.

* 2 cups of carrots.

* 2 sundried tomatoes, soaked.

* 1 strip of seaweed (such as dulse), soaked.

Finely chop the seaweed and garlic, then mince or blend everything.

Warm Feeling Inside Salad
Shazzie says: "This salad is such a comforting one, it will make you glow!"

* 1 lettuce.

* 1 or 2 fennel bulbs (depending on size).

* 1 red onion.

* 1 clove of garlic.

* 1 red pepper, de-seeded.

* 1 orange pepper, de-seeded.

* 6 tomatoes.

* 1 cup of pumpkin sprouts or seeds, soaked.

* 4 sticks of celery.

* 2 avocados, peeled and stoned.

* 10 macadamias.

* 1 cup of watercress.

* 4 dates, stoned.

Prepare the lettuce in your favourite way, chop the fennel, onion, peppers, tomatoes, watercress and celery. Finely chop the garlic and dates, and slice the avocado. Toss all the ingredients together except the macadamias – you need to throw these on top from a very great height.

Sunset Pudding

* 2 bananas, peeled.

* 1 mango, skinned and stoned.

* 10 strawberries.

* 2 dates, stoned (optional, because this is a very sweet pudding).

Chop the dates. Put everything in a food processor and blend, or blend by hand, until it looks like a pudding.

SOME OTHER SAVOURY DISHES FROM STEVE'S FRIENDS
One thing to note in raw recipes is that adding lemon juice, as well as bringing out flavours, is good because it helps prevent oxidation of foods.

Cold pressed olive oil and salty flavours are also often helpful in making a transition from a normal diet to one which is 'high raw'. Apple cider vinegar is a great alternative to lemon juice, particularly for temperate or cooler climates.

The Famous Raw Chickpea Humous
Organic dried Chickpeas, soaked overnight and then left to sprout for between 1 and 3 days starts this off. Using either a hand mincer or a blender the core ingredients are chickpeas and garlic, and some water if I'm using the blender. That's the base and it doesn't necessarily need anything else added. However, depending on what I have available, whose kitchen I'm in and who I'm preparing it for (i.e. those who are on a 'normal' diet tend to want a bit more of the salty flavours) I might add lemon juice and/or cold pressed olive oil (brings the flavour up and out)— with the chickpeas and garlic this is the basic delicious raw humous and it really does not need anything; so try it like this first before experimenting with other tastes.

Other tastes you can add to the humous:

* Salty element (desirable for many, but not essential): celery or chard stalks, seaweed, dried tomatoes, miso, tamari – or if you are still using salt then good quality seasalt.

* Seeds: linseed/flax, ground sesame (not soaked before hand), sunflower, hemp, pumpkin (ideally soaked before hand) – or if you prefer you can add tahini (ideally raw, but which normally is difficult to obtain raw).

* Chopped herbs to mix in or sprinkle on top when blended or minced.

* Chilli (preferably fresh raw or sundried), ginger or other hot ingredients to spice it up when I feel like it.

* Finely chopped Tomato and/or onion can be added on some days.

* Sometimes, if I'm a bit low on chickpeas and it needs filling out, or if I fancy a flavour change, I might add some carrot, squash/pumpkin or parsnip.

* And dried *Ginkgo biloba* leaves (harvested from the local park and dried oneself ideally!) – a very beneficial herb for the brain and circulation, but which is certainly not an essential ingredient.

This humous is great as a basic, delicious, variable and cheap base for salads in cooler climates, where avocados (which are another favourite base for salad dishes) might be out of the price range and ecologically less desirable (due to their embodied 'food miles'). The humous is also great with dips, and in raw 'salad sandwiches', heaped into a large cabbage leaf, spinach leaf, lettuce leaf or chard leaf.

The Turner's Field T'rific Green Salad

The idea behind this recipe is that once you've read this book you'll go out and make sure you have a whole lot of these plants growing happily in your garden, allotment, window box, a friend or relative's garden which is happy to have received some loving attention from you, a nearby hedgerow or any place you can get your hands on. This salad involves walking round the garden, preferably barefoot, picking all or any of the following that can be combined into a green salad of unbelievable vibrancy and deliciousness! It's also great to take children round to help you, giving them the chance to taste (with care, as some tastes are strong) and see each of the plants as you go:

✱ Rocket, perpetual spinach, perennial onion leaves, perennial or annual broccoli (leaves and/or sprouts), perennial or annual kale, chives, lemon balm, sorrel, landcress, lovely lovage, parsley, *Peltaria*/garlic cress, campanula, sweet cicely, fennel, thyme, garlic chives, leek leaves, dandelions, with some finely chopped sage or rosemary, and if its spring or early summer ransoms and hedge garlic (Jack-by-the-Hedge), oriental salad leaves and so on. That's what I call a salad! And if you want a lettuce then one of the best I have found is Black Seeded Simpson's – seeds available from Future Foods, who, like the Agroforestry Research Trust, also supply seeds for loads of great salad plants.

The final vital and vibrant ingredient that gives it that beautiful Turner's Field touch is a few (or loads!) of what ever flowers are available: borage, calendula, chives, mallow, lavateria, nasturtiums, and so on. There is nothing quite like a flower-festooned salad to bring beauty to the meal.

Ariadne's Wolf-Up

This is a serious power-pack of a dish, and is a favourite of Ariadne Fern (of the project Plants for a Future), who is a trained nutritionist. It is also one of my own favourites and really gives me a feeling of vitality and strength. It is designed to be packed with chlorophyll as well as including seeds that contain particular 'essential' amino acids. For many people early on it is worth trying – and for some people you may need to adjust to the new diet before you get a taste for it. Wolf-up involves picking a lot of wild greens and salad greens and then putting these through a hand mincer (some of which look like a wolf's head in profile, hence the name). Add to the greens ground hemp, sunflower, pumpkin and/or flax seeds, and some lemon juice and garlic if required. Some celery or chard stems will add a 'salty' element to the flavour. If you find it too powerful to start with try less wild greens – it's worth experimenting as it's a dish that really grows on you.

Guacamole

Very popular – avocados mashed or blended with a range of other ingredients: garlic and lemon juice are the two basic essentials, although finely chopped tomato and onion/chives are also often added. I find that adding different herbs like dill, parsley and coriander/cilantro on different occasions adds to the fun of experimenting with dishes that are always delicious anyway! A bit of chilli and/or ginger gives it some extra zing if you like it like that. Have it with a big salad of mixed leaves.

January's Sprouted Quinoa Salads

This particular January is not the month, she is a very lively long term raw food chef and teacher living near Stroud (UK). And she does some amazing things with her sprouted Quinoa! Quinoa is one of those fantastic foods that most people think you have to cook; but you don't. Soak it for a few hours, or overnight, then drain it off and then you'll almost be able to watch those little sprouts grow before your eyes. Rinse and drain them once a day, and they are ready from 2 to 4 days.

January's Quinoa salads vary enormously and are always delicious: tomato, a little red onion, some seaweed, celery, a little lemon juice, some fresh herbs... what ever takes your fancy. The great thing about sprouting Quinoa (organic of course) is that it is so simple, quick and cheap, and a totally reliable basis for a sprouted salad. And this dish is a perfect example of how one person's creativity can spark off a wide range of joyful eating experiences for many others.

Chris' Raw Curry

Another example of one person's creativity, this is normally a real eye-opener and taste-teaser for normal eaters and raw foodies alike. A genuine tasting, delicious raw curry... wow!

* Curry ingredients: avocado, red or other onions (according to your taste preferences), carrots, some cauliflower stem, some soaked dates (make a real difference), lemon juice, and what ever else you feel like throwing in – chopped as necessary. Fresh coconut, or organic creamed coconut (which the manufacturers tell us is not heat treated) is a great addition too, that really takes this dish into another dimension.

* Spices and flavour: cumin seeds (the key to the genuine curry flavour), curry powder, ginger, garlic, chilli, cayenne, etc.

* Raw 'Rice' base: cauliflower, chopped very fine or put through a hand mincer or food processor.

Mix or hand mince the main curry ingredients, spices and flavours together, ideally by hand-mincer or using a food processor rather than a blender, so that you have lots of chunky bits. Finely chop the cauliflower using a hand-mincer or food processor, or finely chop by hand, to create the fine white 'rice' bed and then serve the curry on top or at the side, with other side dishes and garnished as you wish. It looks great and it's delicious!

Amanda's Sweet (not hot) Curry Sauce

Blend or hand mince together tomatoes, carrots or pumpkin/squash, olive oil, desiccated coconut or some creamed coconut block (not a whole block!), mild curry powder and other curry spices and / or a little garlic if you wish.

Dao's Seed Paté

There are a number of variations on the basic seed paté recipe. Soaked seeds are best, which usually will be organic hemp, sunflower or pumpkin, all or any of them. These should be put through the hand grinder or mincer, or the blender. Ground dry linseed/flax seeds are good addition which will thicken up the blend, and of course sesame can be used too. If you haven't soaked your main seed ingredients then dry seeds can be put through a seed grinder, hand or electric. To these can be added a whole bunch of other ingredients, with the two keys being lemon juice to bring up the flavour and prevent oxidation, and a salty element, which may be any of those mentioned in the Humous recipe above.

You should not use more than 100 grammes (3-4 ounces) or so of seeds per person, so it works well to add in the minced vegetables with the seeds to bulk it up. These additional ingredients can include fresh or dried herbs, tomatoes, red peppers, onion, mushrooms and all sorts of other ingredients... including chilli or ginger to spice it up if you like that. Add any more liquid elements carefully so that the paté does not get sloppy*. These ingredients can be put through a hand mincer if you've got one, or you can use what ever food processor works for you. The main thing is to experiment, and then you'll find and be able to produce your own favourite paté mixes.

* Ground Linseed is a great ingredient to use to thicken up savoury or sweet dishes alike, if they get a bit sloppy.

Falafel Patties

This one is a minor adaptation from Frederic Paténaude's recipe book *Sunfood Cuisine* – one of the best that's available for raw 'haute cuisine'. It is a favourite dish that is expertly produced by Joe and Carme, great raw friends of Ecoforest, who live nearby.

❋ 1.5 cups of sprouted lentils or chick peas.

❋ 1 cup sprouted sunflower seeds.

❋ 1 tablespoon minced garlic.

❋ 2 cups fresh cilantro/coriander, chopped (or a tablespoon in powder form).

❋ 1/2 cup fresh parsley.

❋ 1/2 cup sesame seeds (or raw tahini).

❋ Salty element according to taste, not too much though (seaweed, minced or chopped chard stalks or celery).

❋ 1/2 cup chopped onion.

❋ 1/2 cup freshly squeezed lemon juice.

❋ 1/4 cup olive oil.

❋ 1.5 teaspoons ground cumin seed, or powder.

Combine all ingredients using a hand mincer or blender, and then have fun forming a blended mixture into small patties. Leave them in a sunny or warm place (ideally in direct sunlight) to dry for up to 8 hours.

Other Great Salad Dishes

✳ One great secret is to use large spring cabbage, kale or white cabbage leaves or other large leaves such as spinach, lettuce or chard if you like it – most of which are easy to grow. These are great for making raw 'tacos' or real 'salad sandwiches' – just fill them with what ever dishes or dips you've got on the table, roll it up and enjoy the experience!

✳ Grated carrot with orange and ginger makes a great combination of flavours.

✳ Raw grated beetroot/beets is fantastic as it is, or with just a dash of lemon juice or apple cider vinegar; beetroot/beet is easy to grow in a good rich soil.

✳ Surprisingly perhaps, grated parsnip with some chopped leek, green onions or plenty of chives, with or without a little lemon juice and olive oil is fantastic; parsnips can be a great root vegetable to grow as a self-seeder, chives and perennial onions are easy too, and leeks are not too much trouble.

✳ Experiment (but do not go over-board) with seed dips. Soak seeds over night (Sunflower, hemp, etc.) and then blend them with some water and various flavours and vegetables to create a mix of tastes (garlic, tomato, red pepper, herbs such as dill, lemon juice, carrot, etc.).

✳ Celery stems, and sliced carrot, cucumber or courgette/zucchini are great for dipping into the raw humous, guacamole, paté or seed dips mentioned above – zucchini and celery are relatively easy to grow, whilst cucumbers can require a bit more attention and carrots do best in certain soils (loose/rich/sandy).

✳ Sprouted green lentils–so easy, so cheap to produce organically, and so delicious. Just soak them overnight, rinse them once a day, and then they are ready from the second or more usually the third day onwards. They are a great and simple basic sprout, that I find simpler and more tasty than many others. Chick peas are equally easy and delicious, and a great sprout if you like something to get your teeth into.

Some More Sweet Dishes

If you are trying to encourage a health creating diet, then knowing a few good raw sweet dishes is especially good for children... big and small! At the same time, recognise that these dishes are transition dishes. They should not be used to reinforce unhealthy patterns of behaviour, like rewards for being good, when they in themselves are not such healthy food combinations. The very best sweet dishes are the simplest – sweet fruits on their own!

Devin's Pie

Like Chris's Curry, the legend of Devin's Pie has spread fast! This is great fun to make because you get to lick all the sweet stickiness of the dates off your fingers! Essential ingredients:

* Dates and almonds are best for the base, sunflower seeds are good too, although other nuts and seeds can be added.
* Various fruits for the filling, with avocado and banana being great staples for this. Fruits that are 'pretty' either sliced or whole to place on the surface (kiwi, apple, orange, strawberry, grapes, raspberries, etc.).

Mince and mix the dates and almonds (preferably soaked beforehand) in either a hand mincer or a food processor; various other nuts and seeds can be added, such as sunflower, hemp, walnuts, linseed, etc. This creates a sticky base that is then pressed firmly into a dish (very lightly running over the dish with avocado or cold pressed olive oil before will help when trying to lift this sticky base out when serving it!).

Then blend or mash up the fruit filling but keep the avocado separate, mixing it with some lemon juice. Blend together all or any of the following: banana, pear, apple, mango, cherimoya (if you are lucky enough to have them available), and so on. If you can finely grind some linseed, then mix this in, this will help to thicken up the filling (and if added to the base it will help bind that too, but it is not essential). Pour this fruit mix into the base first, then spread the mashed avocado layer on top of it.

Slice the 'pretty' fruits finely and lay them on top of the fruit filling to finish off; one or several carefully placed flowers will also add to the 'wow' factor when its brought on to the table. You might need to keep a second one hidden away just in case your life's in danger for not providing second helpings...! You can try all sorts of fruit mixes, including more temperate mixes – to create blackberry and apple pie for example or a summer soft fruit pie. Hazel nuts and walnuts can be used as a base also.

Sibila's Sublime Birthday Cake
Mix together tahini, fresh orange juice, chopped dates, carob powder, some crushed or broken walnut pieces, and then ground sunflower seed and ground linseed to thicken it up. Other nut butters can also be added if you want it even more super rich than it is already. Banana can also be used in the mix. You can have it as a cake or roll it into balls, perhaps rolled in carob powder or finely grated coconut. If it's served as a cake then thin slices of fruit like orange, banana, kiwi or apple can be added to beautify the surface. But remember dishes like this are just for birthdays and special occasions don't make them too much of a habit!

Lexi's Green Pudding (*thanks to Tish*)
This is Lexi's pudding in the sense that she loves eating it as well as making it... she was five at the time this was written. It's very simple, and delicious. Just take two avocados, two bananas and the fresh juice of either two oranges or two apples, and blend them all together, dole it out and then eat it. Yum. Oh, yes, and please try to remember to leave some for the kids!

To add an extra dimension to the nutritiousness you can add a spoonful of spirulina. To vary the flavour another option is to add a spoonful of carob powder.

Gaura's Sweet Balls

Soak nuts and seeds (almonds, walnuts, sunflower, etc.) overnight and blend or mince them together mainly with dates, although raisins and dried figs can also be used. Using some unsoaked seeds may help keep the balls firmer. In Spain at Ecoforest we have discovered that adding the flesh of sun-dried ripe black olives adds a remarkably delicious bitter-sweet chocolate effect to these sweet balls; and finely grated or minced carob pods (with the very hard seeds taken out) also add to the deliciousness. Although they're not raw you can add spices like cinnamon, and even organic fair trade cocoa or carob powder to help soften your taste path on the early transition pathway.

I must point out that the sweet dishes that combine many ingredients are not good to eat on a regular basis as they do not represent good combining. Raw cakes, with lots of sweet fruit, seeds and nuts taste great to those accustomed to feeding a typical western appetite, but they certainly do not represent the healthiest way to eat. After a while of eating more healthily you will find out what this means for your body. Most sweet fruits taste best on their own, and to me taste and feel better than any complex cake. It might take you time to adjust of course, but make sure you give yourself the chance to adjust more quickly and more healthily by limiting the complexities. Keeping it simple is best.

Generally when it comes to raw food preparation I encourage you to be adventurous, play and experiment in creating beautiful and delicious dishes. Creating delicious raw meals, whether it's for your daily meals or for a special occasion, is actually much easier than cooking. For more recipes you can contact Ecoforest for our own simple recipe book, or explore the wide variety of recipes in many raw food books available from US and UK raw food networks by mail order (see Appendix 3 for contacts and recipe books).

ALMONDS

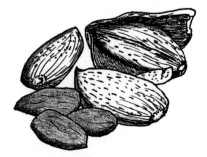

Appendix 2: About Ecoforest

Ecoforest

An ecological vegan raw food forest garden community in southern Spain.

Ecoforest is the only place on the planet that I know of that is experimenting with putting the Working With Nature philosophy into life as fully as possible. We have made a start... and we know that there is still a very long way to go.

Eco Forest Education for Sustainability,[66] which owns the land that is now called Ecoforest, is a not for profit organisation that exists to promote education about simple, natural sustainable living. For us at Ecoforest nature's first law is to work with nature, inside and outside, individually and as a community.

This simple truth, that eating more raw foods offers a route to physical health (when combined with healthy mental attitudes, etc.) and also offers a route to planetary ecological health, is the essence of Ecoforest. We do not suggest that this is a truth for everyone, but it is one we have found to be true for ourselves, and have found works for us.

Ecoforest is a place where people can learn about plants, permaculture, paradise gardening and a healthy, low-impact, affordable and highly sustainable lifestyle. The mass of humanity has become so disconnected from our natural foods, the soil and plants that people need places where they can experience re-connection. So this is what we offer at Ecoforest. Most people (particularly from the so called 'developed' nations) start without a clue about seeds, soil and planting – but they learn fast and they love seeing the constantly amazing results. "Wow, it works! Plants grow! Nature really does know what she's doing! Awesome!"

We have had a constant stream of visitors since we bought the land in August 2000. And they all seem to love it. For those that want to stay or become involved we have a Resident Voluntary Project Worker option and a Visitor option. The former means that after putting down a returnable deposit of four thousand pounds[67], you can live at Ecoforest as part of this amazingly positive project at a very low cost, with a very high quality of life, amongst a group of ecologically minded raw fooders, all working for the common purpose of the project, which is to provide education about sustainable living. One term for this lifestyle is Paradise Gardening... need I say more?!

Another vital element of the Ecoforest vision that we are already putting into practice is living and working in community. This is another one of those natural laws that goes along with diet. Humans are social animals. We don't need to live in each other's pockets but we do need regular and close contact with others, and with nature, for our full physical, mental, emotional

---

[66] As an associated project of the BCM Permaculture Association (Charity No 290897).

[67] Correct at the time of writing – and potentially subject to change.

and spiritual health. It is certainly healthier for us to live in community than it is to live separated lives – living in boxes, travelling in boxes, working in boxes, being buried in boxes! I should qualify that by saying that it is healthier provided you are open to learning how to live in a community. Most of us have learnt survival strategies for living our separated lives – and it can be hard letting go of these and trusting the wider group. So living together again as a community requires some learning, which can be challenging, whilst also being great fun and full of growth. And when I say community I mean like an eco-village or eco-neighbourhood – I do not mean a commune.

At Ecoforest we are keen to help raw vegan eco-communities get going – either following the Ecoforest model and adapting it to local conditions as necessary or by doing it your own way. We've had many American folks over here for example being part of what we're doing because in all the huge diversity and opportunity that America presents they haven't found anything like Ecoforest over there. Well, we can all work together to change that, so let's do it and not hang around.

So our medium term vision is to establish or be well on the way to establishing five other Eco Forest type communities around the world. These need to be on different continents and therefore the USA, South or central America, Asia, Australia and Africa are proposed as locations for this first generation of Eco Forest communities.

And the long term vision for 15 to 25 years is for Eco Forest to become as successful and widespread as McDonalds is now! Personally, I hope that McDonalds will experience a massive decline and reincarnation as something more positive for health and sustainability by 2020. Obviously, I am making a deliberate comparison with McDonalds and other so called 'junk food' providers, and what I might call 'junk drink' providers such as Coca Cola.

At Ecoforest we plan and expect to have a very positive health and environmental impact, rather than us having a negative impact in these areas. We want Ecoforest to be contributing positively to the economy and society, helping to create health and sustainability rather than ill-health and ecological destruction, and to be providing high quality information and education. Because the world seems to me to need many more organisations that are providing health creating food rather than sickness creating foods.

Looking that many years ahead, we want to see most towns with a positive place where people, and particularly children, can visit, and work, live and learn so that they can experience everything they need to about sustainable and healthy living. The Vision is to create innovative and utterly sustainable communities, eco-neighbourhoods and eco-villages, both with land to grow their own food and with places to live and to demonstrate and educate others how to live a sustainable and healthy lifestyle. These eco-neighbourhoods and communities will focus on creating optimal, positive, sustainable, fulfilling ways of living in harmony with the planet by:

* Living and growing organically and ecologically for optimum nutrition and health (human, ecological, body, mind, emotions and spirit) – specifically combining forest/paradise gardening, vegan permaculture and fruit/raw food nutrition.

* Focusing on learning and creativity as naturally complementary themes.

* Creating places and communities for the children – thinking and acting to meet the needs of the adult generations by understanding the needs of the next generation and future generations, thereby freeing the children from the current unsustainable continuum and enabling them to create something new.

* Exploring consciousness, human potential and the experience of being human – researching and exploring consciousness and spirituality[68] as the central problem (solution of human/ecological unsustainability) of sustainability.

By focusing on inter-connectedness, particularly in relation to ecology, nutrition, consciousness, learning and creativity, and the inter-connections between the present and the future through the generations, the project deliberately sets out to move the creative edge of practical living research into healthy and sustainable lifestyles. Instead of having a primary focus on economic growth, the objectives of these communities would be to achieve growth in lifestyles, patterns of thinking and understanding, and patterns of behaviour that are automatically sustainable and health creating. And therefore there is a conscious purpose to create growth in:

* Compassion.

* Fulfilment.

* Love.

* Happiness.

* Wisdom (including wise science and not just clever science).

* Ecological and spiritual understanding.

... and why not?! In due course, health and sustainability will follow as a natural result, as will prosperity. The focus will be on consciously and responsibly meeting our current needs, and the needs of the next and future generations, where our needs are recognised as being physical, social, spiritual, emotional, and intellectual.

Ecological and raw food communities are an essential part of a successful vision of the future, because there are two things that need healing – the inter-related human body, mind and spirit, and this amazing planet that is our home. And who knows, once we have consciously acted to implement that healing process we may just find that those two things are not in fact two, but one after all... Working with nature – it's great! Contact details for Ecoforest see Appendix 3.

---

[68] Just in case any one is worried, this vision does not involve a religion, or involve developing some cult or other. It does involve us being aware that we are conscious beings, with many 'inner' dimensions for us to experience and explore.

Appendix 3: Useful Contacts and Information

For excellent advice on the vast range of tasty raw edibles contact Plants for A Future for their information sheets on edible fruits, salad gardens, perennials, etc. Patrick Whitefield's minimalist garden sections in back issues of *Permaculture Magazine* are very useful, as are his books (see below). Keep Robert Hart and Graham Bell's books close at hand, and you can also visit the PFAF and Permaculture Home Pages on 'the Web'.

LIVING/RAW FOODS CONTACTS AND INFORMATION

Ecoforest: Apdo. 29, Coin 29100, Malaga, Spain. Web: www.ecoforest.org Email: info@ecoforest.org Also www.rawcommunities.com

LIVING/RAW FOODS NETWORKS AND ORGANISATIONS

UK

For information on natural foods/fruit/raw foods in your diet contact:

The FRESH Network and *Get Fresh Magazine*: P.O. Box 71, Ely, Cambridgeshire. CB7 4GU. Tel: 0870 800 7070. Email: karen@fresh-network.com Web: www.fresh-network.com

Elaine Bruce: 49 Gravel Hill, Ludlow, Shropshire SY8 1QS. For Living Foods courses. Tel: 01548 875 308. Email: elaine@livingfoods.enta.net

USA/North America

Frederic Paténaude's sites include information on the excellent magazine *Just Eat An Apple* and Fred's excellent book *Raw Secrets* – spanning North America and with a global interest. Webs: www.sunfood.net and www.rawvegan.com

Dr Douglas Graham, President of Healthful Living International. Dr Graham is an international authority on athletic performance and living foods nutrition. Web: www.doctorgraham.cc

David Klein, Editor of the excellent *Living Nutrition* magazine. PO Box 256, Sebastopol, CA 95473. Web: www.livingnutrition.com

Healthful Living International involves Dr Douglas Graham, Dave Klein, Dr Vivian Vetrano, Prof. Rosalind Gruben and others – an amazing combination of knowledge and experience. Web: www.healthfullivingintl.org

Gabriel Cousens M.D., Director of the Tree of Life Rejuvenation Centre, AZ – living foods with a medical background and a spiritual dimension; author of a number of books. Web: www.treeoflife.nu

Paul Nison, New York, NY – dynamic author of *The Raw Life* and *Raw Knowledge*. Web: www.rawlife.com

Nature's First Law and David Wolfe, San Diego, CA. Dave is one of the most dynamic of raw food advocates and is a great motivational speaker, author of

Sunfood Diet Success System and *Eating for Beauty*, and co-author of *Nature's First Law*. Webs: www.rawfood.com and www.davidwolfe.com – the suppliers of the most complete range of raw food books and products in the world.

Dr Joel Robbins, medical practitioner with excellent *Health Through Nutrition* and *Attitudes to Health* tapes (the best general introduction I've found yet) and books on raw/living foods nutrition: Health Dynamics Corp., 6711 South Yale, Suite 106, Tulsa, Oklahoma 74136. Tel: 1 800 653 5444.

Reverend George Malkmus, Hallelujah Acres, USA – 'pioneering the Christian/ biblical truth of a natural diet and way of life' – author of *Why Christians Get Sick* and *God's Way to Health*.

International Raw & Living Foods Association and Annual Raw & Living Foods Festival (in Portland) the biggest raw event of the year – 8700 SW Borders, Portland, OR 97223. Web: www.rawfoods.com/festival

US RAW FOOD MAGAZINES

Just Eat An Apple (JEAA), editor Fred Paténuade, USA/Can. Webs: www.sunfood.com or www.rawvegan.com

Living Nutrition, editor Dave Klein. Web: www.livingnutrition.com – superb!

SOME OTHER INTERNATIONAL RAW FOODS CONTACTS

Fruitarian Network News, Australia – raw vegan network and magazine. PO Box 293, Trinity Beach, QLD 4879, Australia. Web: www.livingnutrition.com/fwn

R.E.A.L. News, Australia – non-vegan raw magazine.

Die Wurzel network, congresses and magazine, Wurzel-Gesundheitsforum: Excellent raw food and natural living network, with two annual 'congresses' in summer (a large, international event with around 250 attendees each day in 2002, and an excellent range of speakers) and winter. Michael Delius, Torworststrasse 22, 90480 Nurnberg, Germany. Web:www.die-wurzel.de

Naturlich Leben (magazine)/Bund Fur Gesundheit E., V Talstrasse 36, D – 52525 Heinsberb, Germany. The president is Franz Konz, the most wellknown German raw food authority – easily found via the internet.

Naturaleza Cruda, Balta, Lista De Correos, Monda, (Malaga), Spain – text now in both Spanish and English.

Sibila, Finca Amor y Vida, Apdo 73, El Escorial 28280, (Madrid), Spain.

Other international contacts and networks are available from The FRESH Network, Nature's First Law or Living Nutrition, as well as other sources.

LIVING/RAW FOOD READING

Available with many others from the FRESH Network Book Service, Living Nutrition or Nature's First Law – addresses as above:

Raw Secrets, by Frederic Paténaude (ISBN 09 7309300 5), editor of *Just Eat An Apple* magazine and author of *Sunfood Quisine*. *Raw Secrets* is my strongest recommendation for those wanting a very straight-forward handbook on the pros and cons of raw foods, with particularly honest attention to the mistakes that some people commonly make.

Books by Dr Douglas Graham, leading international athletic performance trainer and nutritional adviser, and President of Healthful Living International: *On Nutrition and Physical Performance: A Handbook for Athletes and Sports Enthusiasts* is a really excellent bbok, which is very simple and clear, and is definitely not just for athletes but for anyone who wants to be fit and healthy, and who wants to understand how some of the key processes in our body work without over-complicated explanations – also *Grain Damage* on the significant physically and environmentally damaging effects of large scale grain consumption – and *The High Energy Diet Recipe Guide*.

Raw Life and *Raw Knowledge* by Paul Nison – Paul has probably been the most active person in awakening New York and the east coast of the USA to the huge benefits of eating more raw foods, and the practicalities of transition – his books make inspiring and practical reading.

The Sunfood Diet Success System by David Wolfe – which is continuing to have a huge impact, and which is a raw best seller. Also by David Wolfe *Eating For Beauty*, and *Nature's First Law*, with Steven Arlin and RC Dini.

Intuitive Eating by Susie Miller and Karen Knowler, The Women's Press, London, 2000. About allowing the body's wisdom to guide your diet.

Conscious Eating and *The Rainbow Diet* by Dr Gabriel Cousens – a fabulous 'bible' for those used to an ayurvedic perspective, as well as those wanting a more spiritual approach.

Cooking With Mother Nature by Dick Gregory – a great raw starter for blokes/ guys in particular with plenty of information, humour and feeling.

The New Raw Energy by Leslie and Susannah Kenton, Vermilion, London, 1994 – a good raw starter.

The Next Step by Aranya – for anyone looking into raw issues, available online: www.aranyagardens.co.uk/Diploma Portfolio/Supplementary/Next Step.htm

Health Through Nutrition audio tape by Dr. Joel Robbins – superb, and packed with brilliantly presented information and advice – just get it! (see contact details above)

Loren Lockman, booklets and tapes, available via The Tanglewood Wellness Centre website.

Children of the Sun by Gordon Kennedy – a really wonderful and inspiring book that's not about food! It's about the people of the raw and natural living movement and its European and US origins.

Franz Konz, a wide range of books in German, including the German raw food 'bible' *Der Grosse Gesundheits* – Konz and others are available from Die Wurzel.

Franz Konz is also president of *Naturlich Lieben* raw foods and natural living magazine which also supplies a wide range of books. Web: www.die-wurzel.de

Balta, editor of *El Boletin* magazine, now produced with text in both Spanish and English. A wide range of books in Spanish is also available. Balta: Lista de Correos, Monda, Provincia de Malaga, Spain.

Sibila's (previously Nuria Aragon Castro) first book: *Vida Libre y Natural: en el sendero de la sencillez y el amor* (Free and Natural Life: on the trail of simplicity and love) includes chapters on the simple raw vegan nutrition, home education, not vaccinating, and several other fascinating elements on the pathway of a truly free and natural life (published in Spanish by Mandala Ediciones, Madrid, 2002. ISBN 84 95052 82 0).

Jose Manuel Casada Sierra – *Las Frutas, Nuestro Alimento Ideal*, Higea, Colmenar Viejo (Madrid) Spain. An excellent Spanish raw food book, with recipes and a great deal of information. ISBN 84 88722 095.

RAW RECIPE BOOKS

Sunfood Cuisine by Frederic Paténaude.

The Raw Gourmet by Nomi Shannon.

Living Nutrition's Favourite Alive Raw Food Recipes compiled by Dave Klein.

The High Energy Diet Recipe Guide by Dr Douglas Graham.

Other raw food books that include a large number of recipes:

The Sunfood Diet Success System and *Eating for Beauty* by David Wolfe.

RAW PARENTING

Information sources and books to help parents and children are growing all the time now – these are designed to help with less than 100% raw lifestyles and transitioning, as well those that wish to create a 100% raw lifestyle. Some of the excellent resources that are now available include:

The Boutenko Family (US) – and *Raw Family*: a true story of awakening. Web: www.rawfamily.com

Raw Kids by Cheryl Stoykoff – transitioning kids to a raw food diet. Web: www.livingspiritfoundation.org

Get Fresh magazine, Fresh Network UK has a regular raw parenting column.

The Continuum Concept by Jean Liedloff, Perseus Books. A really important book, although not about diet or nutrition.

Primal Mothering in a Modern World, Hygeia Halfmoon.

The Mother Magazine: Veronica Robinson, The Cottage, Glassonby, near Penrith, Cumbria CA10 1DU, UK. Web: www.themothermagazine.co.uk Excellent on natural mothering.

OTHER CONTACTS FOR ELEMENTS OF WHOLE HEALTH

Meditation: Transcendental Meditation and Vipassana can be found through the internet, as can the Federation of Western Buddhists.

Yoga and Tai Chi: *The Five Tibetans*, Christopher Kilham, Healing Arts Press, 1994 – also *Just Eat An Apple*, Jan-Feb 2001 edition (issue 15) for an excellent summary of '*The Five Tibetans*'/'*The Tibetan Rites*' by Frederic Paténaude. There are many useful books on yoga and tai chi – the best thing is to go out and find a teacher, and take a course, then continue the practice yourself regularly either independently or within a local group/group of friends.

Ki Aikido: Enquiries verbally or via www.Ki-aikido.net (USA) or www.Kifedgb. force9.co.uk (UK) will find a local or regional teacher, or course.

Artistic, voice-work and creative endeavours: there are many books and courses available to help you express your creative side in a healthy and spiritually positive way – *The Artist's Way* by Julia Cameron and *The Healing Voice* by Paul Newham are examples that several friends have found very useful.

Community, group work and communication: *Creating Harmony* edited by Hildur Jackson, Permenant Publications is a great book on the lessons and practicalities of community living – drawing on examples of communities world-wide, with most sections written by members of those communities. The *North America Communities* magazine is excellent; 138-PA Twin Oaks Road, Louisa, VA 23093; Tel: 800 462 8240 – in the UK and Europe; *Diggers and Dreamers* and *Ecotopia* are excellent directories of intentional communities both available via Permanent Publications. Many courses, organisations and networks can help develop an understanding of our failures and successes in communication, and develop communication skills. The books *Transformations* and *Frogs Into Princes* by J Grinder and R Bandler are excellent guides to understanding and significantly improving communication, as is *Non Violent Communication* – www.cnvc.org and www.LifeResouces.co.uk

PERMACULTURE INFORMATION AND CONTACTS
Permaculture Networks and Organisations

USA Contacts

Permaculture Activist: PO Box 1209, Black Mountain, NC 28711, USA. Web: www.permacultureactivist.net

American Permaculture Directory: John Irwin, Pennsylvania. Email:jwirwin@permaculture.net

Permaculture Institute USA: Scott Pitman, New Mexico. Email: pci@permaculture-inst.org

Central Rocky Mountain Permaculture Institute: Web: www.crmpi.org

Earthaven Ecovillage: Culture's Edge, 1025 Camp Elliot Rd, Black Mountain, NC 28711. Web: www.earthaven.org

Joe Hollis, Mountain Gardens, 3020 White Oak Creek Road, Burnsville, NC 28714. Web: http://webpages.charter.net/czar207196/garden.htm

UK Contacts

BCM Permaculture Association: London WC1N 3XX. Tel: 01654 712 188. Email: office@permaculture.org Web: www. permaculture.org

Permanent Publications: The Sustainability Centre, East Meon, Hampshire GU32 1HR. Tel: 0845 458 4150 (UK local rate) or +44 1730 823 311 (International). Email: enquiries@permaculture.co.uk Web: www.permaculture.co.uk

VON (Vegan Organic Network): Anandavan, 58 High Lane, Chorlton, Manchester M21 9DZ. Web: www.veganvillage.co.uk/vohan/index.htm

Plants For A Future: PFAF, Research Centre and Demonstration Gardens, Blagdon Cross, near Holsworthy, Devon. Tel: 0845 458 4719 (UK local rate). Web:www.comp.leeds.ac.uk/pfaf/

Australian Contacts

Djanburig Gardens PC Education Centre: Nimbin, NSW. Email: permed @nor.cor.au Web: www.earthwise.org.au

Permaculture Institute: 31 Rulla Road, Sisters Creek, Tasmania 7325. Email: tagariadmin@southcom.com.au

SEED International: 50 Crystal Waters, Kilroy Lane, Conondale, QLD 4552. Email: info@permaculture.au.com Web: www.permaculture.au.com

Excellent Temperate Climate Resources *(e.g. for Europe and N America)*

Agroforestry News: Agroforestry Research Trust, 46 Hunters Moon, Dartington, Totnes, Devon TQ9 6JT – UK based, but relevant and invaluable for all temperate climate areas. Email: mail@agroforestry.co.uk Web: www.agroforestry.co.uk

Growing Green International: Vegan Organic Network, Anandavan, 58 High Lane, Chorlton, Manchester MZ1 9DZ – international magazine on vegan organic agriculture, horticulture and permaculture.

Permaculture Magazine: UK/European Distributors: Permanent Publications, North American Distributors: Disticor Magazine Distribution, 695 Westney Road South, Suite 14 Ajax, Ontario, Canada LIS 6M9.

Permaculture Works: Newsletter of the BCM Permaculture Association.

Permaculture Activist: Post Office Box 1209, Black Mountain, NC 28711, USA, UK/European Distributors: Permanent Publications.

Permaculture Websites

You will find that these websites have many links, and so, quite easily, you will be able to find the relevant organisations, courses, book sources, active groups, and so on relevant to your particular geographical area.

www.crmpi.org – Central Rocky Mountain Permaculture Institute.

www.earthhaven.org – Earth Haven Ecovillage, permaculture based, N Carolina.

www.gaia.org.ar – Argentinian website.

www.permacultura-es.org –Spanish permaculture website.

www.permakultur-akademie.de – the German Permaculture Academy.

www.permacultureactivist.net – *Permaculture Activist*.

www.permaculture.au.com –SEED International – permaculture, sustainability, education and ecological design. Based at Crystal Waters Permaculture Village in Australia.

www.permaculture.co.uk – *Permaculture Magazine* and *Earth Repair Catalogue* plus details of courses, permaculture articles, design bites, contacts etc.

www.permacultureinstitute.com – Permaculture Institute of Northern California.

www.permaculture.net – North American Permaculture.

www.permaculture.org.nz – New Zealand Permaculture Institute.

www.permaculture.org.uk – BCM Permaculture Association, links to numerous UK and international permaculture groups and other projects, courses, activities, resources, etc. see also www.permaculture.org.uk/academy/index.html on permaculture training – internationally relevant, not just for the UK.

Publishers and Mail Order Book Suppliers

www.chelseagreen.com – Chelsea Green Publishing – major US publishers of mainly ecological, sustainable living and now also natural health books.

www.permaculture.co.uk – Permanent Publications – UK publishers of permaculture and other ecological books, including this one, distributors of a wide range of titles by mail order and on-line bookstore.

Permaculture Reading

A huge range of useful books is available by mail order from Permanent Publications (UK), all described in their excellent catalogue *The Earth Repair Catalogue*, and from Chelsea Green (USA) – or from *Permaculture Activist* magazine – addresses as above – or via your local book shop:

Four of the best introductory books for any climate:

An Introduction to Permaculture (228 pages), Bill Mollison and Reny Mia Sley, Tagari Press, and *Permaculture: A Designers' Manual* (576 pages), by Bill Mollison which is the 'bible' of the permaculture movement.

The Basics of Permaculture Design by Ross Mars – an accessible and practical book.

Forest Gardening (Green Books) is THE text book on the subject, and *Beyond The Forest Garden* (Gaia Books) for the background philosophy, both by Robert Hart.

Edible Landscaping by Robert Kourik – this does not cover the design side of permaculture and issues such as water systems, energy and waste, but is great for the gardening side of permaculture.

And some other really excellent books are:

Food For Free by Richard Mabey, Collins, or *Wild Food* by Roger Philips, Pan Books.

How To Grow More Vegetables by John Jeavons, Ten Speed Press.

Plants For A Future by Ken Fern, Permanent Publications – just superb.

Permaculture Plants by Jeff Nugent & Julia Boniface, Sustainable Agriculture Research Institute – excellent for Mediterranean/sub-tropical and tropical climates.

The Permaculture Garden and *The Permaculture Way* by Graham Bell, Permanent Publications – for an excellent overall perspective.

The Earthcare Manual, How To Make A Forest Garden and *Permaculture In A Nutshell* by Patrick Whitefield, Permanent Publications – extremely practical, packed with information, written by Britain's leading permaculture teacher.

A Handful of Seed and Plant Suppliers
The best source for a list of good seed, plant and tree suppliers is an up-to-date copy of *Permaculture Magazine* (UK), or *Permaculture Activist* (USA) – see addresses and contact details above for a copy by post, if you do know of a local outlet. The following is a small list of suppliers compiled from my own knowledge, and excellent information provided in *Permaculture Magazine*, and *The Permaculture Activist* (Issue 48, article by Suzanne P DeMuth):

The Agroforestry Research Trust (UK, and will supply to many other countries) – supplying seeds and plants – absolutely excellent and large range from trees, to shrubs, to ground cover plants and climbers: 46 Hunters Moon, Dartington, Totnes, Devon TQ9 6JT, UK. Web: www.agroforestry.co.uk

Plants For A Future – particularly for perennials and interesting food and other useful plants, NOT seeds: PFAF, Research Centre and Demonstration Gardens, Blagdon Cross, near Holsworthy, Devon, UK. Tel: 0845 458 4719. And their excellent website at: www.comp.leeds.ac.uk/pfaf/

Future Foods – excellent range of interesting, and in some cases unusual seeds – particularly for salads: PO Box 1564, Wedmore, Somerset BS28 4DP, UK.

Cool Temperate – particularly good for trees and fruit bushes: Newhouse Farm, Kniveton, Ashbourne, Derbyshire DE6 1JL, UK. Tel: 01335 347 067.

Vida Verde (UK and Spain) – A variety of interesting vegetables for both temperate and warmer climates. Buzon 6, Rio de Aguas, Sorbas, 04270 Almeria, Espana and 14 Southdown Avenue, Lewes, East Sussex BN7 1EL. England. Web: www.vidaverde.co.uk Email: info@vidaverde.co.uk

Chase Organics – linked with HDRA, Chase supply a large range of vegetable and herb seeds: River Dene Estate, Molesey Road, Hersham, Surrey KT12 4RG, UK. Tel: 01932 253 666. Web: www.chaseorganics.co.uk

Seed Savers International and Seed Savers Exchange (SSE), 3076 North Winn Rd., Decorah, IA 52101, USA. SSE is the leading US heirloom seed conserving organisation – a non-profit network of around 8,000 members. It maintains a seed bank of 18,000 vegetable varieties at its headquarters, 700 varieties of apples and 200 varieties of grapes. Also the home of Seed Savers International – saving varieties from areas around the world that are rich in crop diversity.

Permaculture Seed and Plant Exchange, c/o Joe Hollis, Mountain Gardens, 3020 White Oak Creek Road, Burnsville, NC 28714, USA. $7.00/year membership (2002), a group of growers and propagators who share information and plant materials, seeds, etc. Web: www.webpages.charter.net/czar207196/garden.htm

Native Seeds, is one of many excellent US seed suppliers. Native Seeds specialise in seeds for dryer climates, and focus in particular on seeds used by native Americans in the high and low desert areas of the south west USA. 526 N 4th Avenue, Tucson, AZ 85705, USA. Web: www.nativeseeds.org

Bountiful Gardens/Ecology Action, 18001 Shafer Ranch Rd., Willits, CA 95490-9626, USA. Supplies seeds for many vegetables, heirloom varieties and other useful plants.

Eastern Native Seed Conservancy, PO Box 451, 222 Main Street, Great Barrington, MA 01230, USA. – non-profit network conserving a huge variety of food and other useful plant resources. Web: www.berkshire.net/ensc/seedmain.html

Arche Noah, Obere Strasse 40, A-3553 Schiltern, Austria. Modelled on the US Seed Savers Exchange, with 1,600+ members, preserving at least 3,000 heritage vegetables, and serving German speaking countries. Linked with Seed Savers International.

Australia: I have not been able to research Australian seed suppliers much but with the highly developed nature of permaculture networks and projects in Australia if you contact local or national permaculture networks and organisations then you will quickly find your way to a wide range of excellent seed suppliers (see Australian PC contacts and websites). Two useful organisations are:

Seed Savers Network/Seed Aid Trust, Box 975, Byron Bay, NSW 2481. Australia – Australia's most developed seed saving organisation, also working in other countries around the world: vegetables, herbs, permaculture plants and fruit trees. Web: www.pm.com.au/seedsave

Heritage Seed Curators Association (HSCA), PO Box 1450, Bairnsdale, Victoria 3875, Australia. Non-profit organisation conserving a wide variety of Australia's horticultural and garden heritage plant resources, mainly vegetables with some fruit.

Generally you should feel confident that through internet searches you will be able to find an excellent range of organic and specialist seed and plant suppliers.

THE FOOD SYSTEM, ECONOMY, SUSTAINABILITY AND THE MEDICAL SYSTEM

Bringing The Food Economy Home by Norberg-Hodge, Merrifield and Gorelick (Zed Books) – local alternatives to global agri-business and the wholesale economic, social and environmental destruction it wreaks.

The Food System by Tansey and Worsley (Earthscan) is an excellent book on the realities of the food sytem and economy from global to local level.

The Earth Dweller's Guide to Sustainability by Steve Charter provides a fascinating and unique perspective on sustainability issues, looking at the background, 'economy – society – environment' and 'civilisastions – consciousness – the individual', along with practical, conscious responses (contact Steve via Ecoforest, Email: info@ecoforest.org).

Dead Doctors Don't Lie (book and tape) by Dr Joel Wallach provides an apparently objective perspective on the effectiveness (or lack of it) of the modern western medical system, and its overall health impacts, costs, etc.

GRAPES

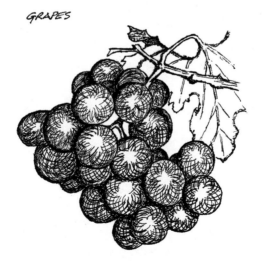

Appendix 4: A Selection of Varieties for Establishing a Forest Garden

The following is a list with some basic information that will help you create an all-year round food producing system. In particular it will be good to start by selecting around 20 to 30 perennial salad plants in the herbaceous and ground cover sections to establish an all year salad garden – the perennial kale, broccoli and onions, perpetual spinach and peltaria/garlic cress are highly recommended as core elements in your salad system.

More information is provided for apples and pears as they are most likely to form the skeleton around which a temperate forest garden is created. The lists of plants are by no means exclusive, and in some cases is very limited. This is because much good information on herbaceous plants in general, including self-seeders, 'cut and come agains' and other salad plants, especially those that are easily grown for summer cropping, is contained in various permaculture books; the book *Plants For A Future* by Ken Fern being a particularly superb reference. You will remember more if you research some of these books for suitable plants for your forest garden.

CANOPY TREES

Apples

Apples are the most important fruit for the temperate climate as they are the hardiest fruit and can be stored for use all year. Apples can be grown as: Standards: plant 4.6-6m (15-20ft) apart; Bush trees: plant 2.4-3m (8-10 ft) apart; Cordons: plant 1.2m (4ft) apart at angle of 45 degrees to restrict the flow of sap and therefore growth; and Dwarf Pyramids: plant 1.8-2.1m (6-7ft) apart, which produce most fruit in the shortest time. To make good wood growth and many fruit buds quickly, make a nick just above each bud on the main stem. Then prune the shoots formed back each year to half the new season's growth.

Use of dwarf trees, particularly using Malling root-stocks, has led to a ten fold increase in density of planting, which is very useful for a small forest garden. Dwarf trees bear fruit rather than produce wood, and come more quickly to heavy fruit bearing. Trees on dwarfing root-stock need careful staking as they do not produce such strong roots. A strong stake is needed approx. 0.3m (1ft) from the roots, at a slight angle, with the bark protected from rubbing against the stake in windy weather.

Apples need a soil with humus for moisture retention for the fruit to make a good size. Grass needs suppressing with a good mulch around the tree when planted to reduce competition for nutrients.

Most apples need other varieties for pollination i.e. they do not set fruit with pollen from their own variety. A mix of varieties is therefore good, with edible crab-apples also being excellent pollinators, especially golden hornet. (Good pollinators are marked ++ in the following list.) As for most trees, planting should be in the dormant period between November and the end of March.

Varieties:

July/August: Devonshire Quarendon/Discovery++/George Cave

Sept./October: Ellison's Orange/ James Grieve++/Katja/Katy/Laxton's Fortune/ Bramley**/Allington Pippin/Charles Ross/Sunset/Egremont Russet++/King of Pippins

November/December: Acme /Kidd's Orange/Pitmaston Pine Apple/ Ribston Pippin/Sunset/Ashmead Kernel/Jupiter/Suntan/Winston/Laxton's Superb/Cox's Orange Pippin **

December/January: Court Pendu Plat **/Sturmer Pippin ** /Tydeman's Late Orange **/Golden Delicious **

Edible crab apples (as understorey trees): John Downie/Golden Hornet ++/ Crittendon/Red Glow – excellent for pollination.

Pears

Pears originate from a warmer climate than apples, so require more warmth to ripen properly – hence their use particularly in walled gardens. Like apples they can be grown in standard, bush, pyramid or cordon forms, although they are often best grown in Espalier form along walls, or trained along strong guides (perhaps use Ramie, or other plant fibres!). Pruning and culture is similar to apples. Pollination is also similar to apples.

Varieties:

Early blooming: Clapps' Favourite (earliest fruiting)/Conference/Beurre Superfin/ Durondeau/Louis Bonne/Margeurite Marillat

Mid-Season blooming: William's Bon Chretien/Beurre Bedfor/Packham's Triumph/Glou Morceau

Late blooming: Doyenne du Comice/Improved Fertility/Winter Nelis

Hardy Pears: Beurre Hardy/Jargonelle/Durondeau/Hessle/Glow Red William

Easiest Pears: Conference/Dr Guyot/William's Bon Chretien (will fertilise each other)

Plums

July/August: River's Early Prolific/Opal/Victoria/Coe's Golden Drop

September/October: Marjorie's Seedling

KEY:	## Needs both male and female for pollination
	** Good for storing
	++ Good pollinator
	~ Shade tolerant

Gages

July/August: Denniston's superb/golden gage

Other Fruit

Sea buckthorn (*Hippophae salicifolia* or *Rhamnoides* – medicinally very powerful), hawthorns (*Crataegus* – various varieties, many with excellent and surprising fruits).

Nuts

Walnut: buccaneer/broadview, chestnut: *Castenea mollissima/cretana*, butternuts, shagbark hickory, American oaks, pine nuts: stone pine/Swiss arola pine/Mexican nut-pine

Warmth and sun loving fruit and nuts:

Peaches, apricots, mulberry, brown turkey fig, whitebeam, almonds

Edible Tree Leaves

Lime, *Ginkgo biloba* (for circulation and brain health), hawthorn leaves

Fruiting Climbers

Blackberry, Siberian kiwi ##, NZ kiwi ##, Romanus rosehips, grape: brant vine/*Vitis coignitiae*/strawberry grape

UNDERSTOREY

Shade tolerants include: medlar, juneberry, lime tree leaves, oregon grape (*Mahonia aquifolium/repens*), hazel/filbert, crab apples

Shrubs

Good shade tolerants:

Gooseberry~, loganberry~, Japanese wineberry~, *Eleagnus*, *Rosa rugosa*, raspberry, red/white currants, tayberry, autumn raspberry, mulberry, blackcurrants, Chinese dogwood, thimbleberry, salmonberry

On acid soils, or in containers: blueberry, cowberry, dewberry, saltbush/*Atriplex halimus*.

Herbaceous/Herbs

See *John Evelyn's Acetaria*: a discourse on sallets (first pub'd 1699, facsimile copies printed more recently) for a superb range of herbal 'sallet' plants.

All Year Round Salad Leaves Or Available During The Winter

Three-cornered leek, spinach beet, *Campanula versiculor*, salad burnet, Turkish rocket, alexanders, dandelions, perennial kale, perennial broccoli, hedge garlic, daffodil garlic, wild garlic, Welsh onions, perennial onion, chives, fennel, sweet cicely, alpine dock, lovage, Good King Henry, Polish sorrel, samphire, mitsuba, corn salad, horseradish, tree onions, Welsh onions, landcress, ribbed plantain.

GROUND COVER

All Year Round Salad Leaves Or Available During The Winter

Peltaria alliacea, *Richardia picroides*, sorrel/*Rumex acetosa*, miner's lettuce, ground ivy, hairy bittercress, pink purslane, *Campanula poscharskyana*, *Claytonia virginica*.

Ground Cover Fruit

Wild/alpine strawberries, dewberry, Japanese strawberry – raspberry, *Rubus tricolor*, *Rubus nutans*.

Roots

Onions, parsnip (which can be a good self-seeder), beetroot, Hamburg parsley, radish (black Spanish/Violet de Gournay), salsify, celeriac.

Self-Seeders and Annuals

Rocket, (American) landcress, nasturtium, borage, radish, spinach, pick'n' pluck lettuces.

Squashes and courgettes/zucchini are particularly productive, with many squashes being excellent winter foods that store well. Chilacayote is an amazing plant of this family for both its large fruit which can store for several years (a bit like a marrow/melon cross) and its long distance rambling habit... if you've got the space!

Flowers

There is nothing more beautiful than a salad bowl laden with flowers: amongst those that are both delicious and beautiful are day lily, mallow, rose, chive, onion and garlic family flowers, borage and other herb flowers, milkweeds, yellow asphodel, nasturtium and calendula. Plants For A Future have a great website and book for more information on edible flowers.

Another Useful and Interesting Plant

Nettles, both for fibre and the raw tips, carefully picked with finger and thumb below the first sets of leaves, then rolled between finger and thumb, are delicious, and high in chlorophyl – useful as an early spring source of food.

REFERENCES

Forest Gardening (Green Books) by Robert Hart; *Plants For A Future* (Permanent Publications), by Ken Fern; *How To Make A Forest Garden* (Permanent Publications), by Patrick Whitefield; *Fruit Growing* (Floraprint), by Roy Genders; *The Permaculture Garden* (Permanent Publications), by Graham Bell.

All Year Harvests for Temperate Climates

	JANUARY - APRIL	MAY - JUNE	JULY - AUGUST	SEPTEMBER - OCTOBER	NOVEMBER - DECEMBER
CANOPY	Stored apples and pears, dried fruits and nuts	Dried fruits and nuts	Apples, plums and gages	Apples, pears, plums, walnut, chestnut, butternuts, shagbark, hicory, oaks, pine-nuts	Apples, pears, buckthorns, persimmon
UNDERSTORY	Hawthorn leaves	Juneberry, lime tree leaves	Peach, apricot, mulberry, figs	Oregon grape, crab apple, rowan, hawthorn, hazel	Medlar
CLIMBERS			Blackberry	Kiwis, rosehips, grapes	
SHRUBS		Eleagnus, gooseberries, saltbush	Early raspberries, red and white currants, loganberry, tayberry, gooseberry, blackcurrants, wineberry, saltbush	Late raspberries, dogwood, thimbleberry, salmonberry, saltbush	
HERBACEOUS		Rocket, sorrell, onions, mallows, mitsuba, horseradish, good king henry, dandelions, plantains, fennel, dill, sweet cicely, lovage, campanulas, tomatoes			
		Chives, perennial kale, perennial spinach, perennial broccoli, perennial onions and garlics			
GROUND COVER		Alexanders, sweet cicely, alpine dock, turkish rocket			
		Wild garlic			
		Corn salad			
ROOT CROPS	Beetroot, parsnip, carrot				Beetroot, parsnip, carrot

The table above gives an *indication* of stacking in time and space, primarily *using perennial plants* to achieve an all year raw harvest with a 'skeleton' forest garden system in a temperate climate. Actual seasons will vary according to the varieties chosen, as well as the climate you are in and the micro-climate you can create or take advantage of to extend the season.

Sub-Tropical and Mediterranean Type Climates

The variety of plants and trees that can be grown is phenomenal once you get into warmer climates. The Australian book *Permaculture Plants* provides a lot of useful information including fast growing trees and shrubs that help improve, secure or rehabilitate the soil, as well as many drought tolerant species (e.g. tagasaste, albizia, leucaena). Robert Hart's book *Forest Gardening* has many useful suggestions for forest gardens in warmer climates, and includes more information on vegetables for these climates. *Introduction to Permaculture* also has a great deal of information on useful plants for these climates.

As with a temperate apple orchard it is relatively easy to transform a traditional orange grove (for example) to a much more diverse forest garden. Your choices include the following, some of which can provide crops for 6 to 8 months of the year if different varieties are selected, and/or different plants of the same variety are placed in subtly different micro-climates on site:

✸ Citrus: oranges, tangerines, grapefruit, lemons, ugli fruit and so on.

✸ Peaches, plums, pears, nectarines, kaki/sharon fruit/persimmon, many varieties of grapes, loquat, passion fruit, kiwi, azerole/edible hawthorn, apricots, figs, olives, pomegranite, prickly pear, mulberry, carob and so on.

✸ Avocados, cherimoyas/custard apple, jujube (Chinese date apple), papayas – hardier, non-commercial varieties can be tended through light frosts and will tolerate these once through their first few years. Mangos, banana and many other delicious fruit need to be frost free. Then there's pawpaw, sapodilla, white sapote, pepino, capuli, tamarillo, ice cream bean, various palms, physallis and so on.

✸ Nuts: walnuts, almonds, pecans, chestnuts, pine nuts, etc.

✸ Many, many varieties of melon, including water melon. Cucumbers, numerous squashes, kiwano and a variety of trailing/climbing plants, including courgettes/zuchinni, chilacayote, and tomatoes.

✸ And a huge variety of perennial and annual vegetables, herbs and so on, including excellent seed producing plants such as sunflower. At Ecoforest (southern Spain) we find rocket, spinach, chard, malva, fennel, various herbs, perennial broccoli, nasturtium, kale, wild and perennial onions, and others grow particularly well, with celery (for example) growing very happily under the orange trees.

✸ In tougher spots, drought tolerant soil improvers include tagasaste, leucaena, Ice cream bean, albizias, casaurinas – and many annual soil improving, nitrogen fixing plants such as alfalfa, chickpeas, peanuts, pigeon pea, clovers and other plants, including the so called 'wonder bean' from South America, the macuna bean.

At Ecoforest in Spain we are experimenting with a very wide range of fruits, salad plants and vegetables – trees, shrubs, climbers and lower growing plants that create a highly productive, low maintenance permaculture and forest garden well suited to the Mediterranean climate.

Fruit Harvests in Mediterranean Climates

Fruit	January - March	April - June	July - September	October - December
Avocados	All year			
Lemons	All year			
Oranges		to June		Nov/Dec start
Grapefruits		to June		December start
Manderins	to March			November start
Tangerines	to March			November start
Chirimoyas	to March			October start
Loquats		April to May		
		April to May		
Strawberries		April to June		
		May to June		
		May to June		
		May to June		
Nectarines		April start	to July	
Peaches		April start	to July	
Mulberries		May start	to August	
Melons		May start		to December
Watermelons		May start		to November
Apples			June start	to December
Pears			June start	to December
Grapes			June start	to December
Figs			August start	to November
Mangos			September start	to December
Pomegranites			September start	to December
Kaki				Oct. to Dec.

I thank Juan Ramos of Coin (Malaga), an experienced organic and permaculture grower in southern Spain (Mediterannean climate), for a great deal of the information in the tabulation above.

The table above gives indications of fruiting seasons – exact seasons will vary according to variety, local climate and the microclimate, i.e. the positioning of different varieties of one type of fruit in sunny spots or shady spots will allow you to extend and vary the season of ripening. With Melons and watermelons it can be possible to start the season earlier where the plants are started in a conservatory, polytunnel or some other form of protection and then planted out when it is warm enough. Other vine fruits such as tomatoes and cucumbers can also be grown in this way, and with protection or in frost free climates tomatoes can be grown all year round. Other fruits that can be grown include papaya and bananas where it is warm enough, olives, passion fruit, kiwi (does best with shade), sapote, lucuma, feijoa (pineapple guava), jujube (Chinese date apple), guava (guayava), cactus fruit (prickly pear, chumbo), raspberries and other berries, and many other types of fruit. Nuts that can be grown include almonds, pecans, walnuts, hazel nuts, chestnuts, and where it is warm enough macadamia and pistacio.

Figs

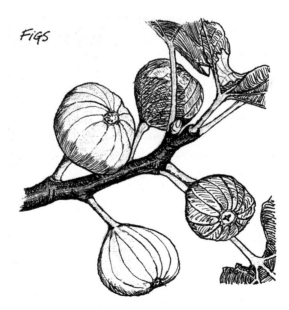

TIPI LIVING

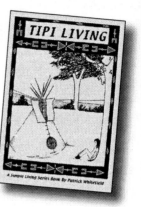

a Simple Living Series book
by Patrick Whitefield
Illustrations by
Anne Monger

Permaculture teacher, Patrick
Whitefield lived in a self built
tipi in Somerset for eight years.
First self-published and now
newly revised and updated,
this is his guide to all aspects
of tipi living: the story of how he came to live this way;
how to choose and pitch a tipi; living with Sun and
Storm; maintenance; moving; firemaking; furnishing;
food and cooking in a tipi. Full of first hand experience
and practical information, it is also Patrick's personal
account of a time of simplicity and spiritual connection
with the Earth. A delightful book for everyone interested
in tipis, low impact dwelling and those who want to
celebrate the simple life.

Permanent Publications; ISBN 1 85623 016 3; A5;
Paperback; 48pp; 35 line drawings; Code TL1; £4.95 + p&p

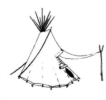

PERMANENT PUBLICATIONS
The Sustainability Centre, East Meon
Hampshire GU32 1HR, UK
Tel: 0845 458 4150 or 01730 823 311
Fax: 01730 823 322
Email: orders@permaculture.co.uk

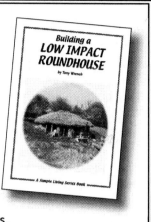
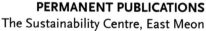

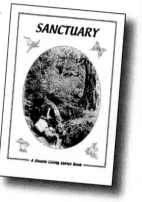